Natural Intelligence

Body-Mind Integration
and Human Development

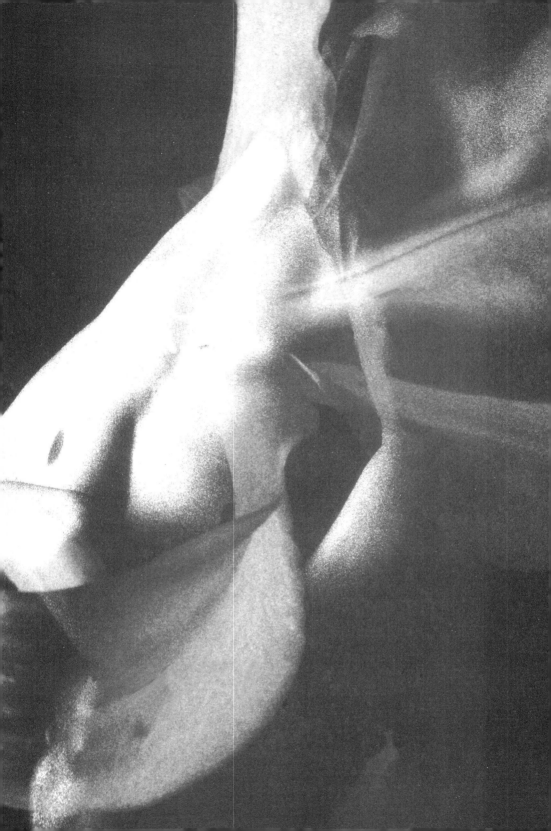

Natural Intelligence

Body-Mind Integration
and Human Development

❋ ❋ ❋

SUSAN APOSHYAN

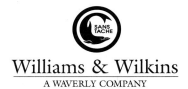

Williams & Wilkins
A WAVERLY COMPANY

BALTIMORE • PHILADELPHIA • LONDON • PARIS • BANGKOK
BUENOS AIRES • HONG KONG • MUNICH • SYDNEY • TOKYO • WROCLAW

Editor: Eric Johnson
Managing Editor: Sue Kimner
Marketing Manager: Chris Kushner

351 West Camden Street
Baltimore, Maryland 21201-2436 USA

The publisher is not responsible (as a matter of product liability, negligence or otherwise) for
any injury resulting from any material contained herein. This publication contains information relating to general principles of medical care which should not be construed as specific in-
structions for individual patients. Manufacturers' product information and package inserts
should be reviewed for current information, including contraindications, dosages and precau-
tions.

Printed in the United States of America

Library of Congress Cataloging-in-Publication Data

Aposhyan, Susan M.
    Natural intelligence: body-mind integration and human development / Susan M.
Aposhyan.
        p.   cm.
    Includes bibliographical references and index.
    ISBN (invalid) 0-683-30559-9
    1. Mind and body.   I. Title.
BF161.A66   1998
150.19′8—dc21   98-26722
                                                                                              CIP

*The publishers have made every effort to trace the copyright holders for borrowed material. If they have
inadvertently overlooked any, they will be pleased to make the necessary arrangements at the first opportunity.*

To purchase additional copies of this book, call our customer service department at **(800) 638-
0672** or fax orders to **(800) 447-8438.** For other book services, including chapter reprints and
large quantity sales, ask for the Special Sales department.

Canadian customers should call **(800) 665-1148,** or fax **(800) 665-0103.** For all other calls
originating outside of the United States, please call **(410) 528-4223** or fax us at **(410) 528-
8550.**

Visit *Williams & Wilkins* on the Internet: http://www.wwilkins.com or contact our customer
service department at **custserv@wwilkins.com.** Williams & Wilkins customer service repre-
sentatives are available from 8:30 am to 6:00 pm, EST, Monday through Friday, for telephone
access.

                                                                              99 00 01 02
                                                                    1 2 3 4 5 6 7 8 9 10

Acknowledgments

I am very blessed to have had two extraordinary teachers in my life, Chogyam Trungpa, Rinpoche and Bonnie Bainbridge Cohen. I thank them each for giving me the means to understand my own vision.

I thank my students, clients, trainees, and colleagues for the constant flow of lively dialogue that has manifested in this book.

I thank my father, Joseph, for bequeathing an earthy, third-world sense of physical play. I thank my mother, Wilma, for teaching me how to think. I thank my brother, Howard, for accompanying me on our parallel paths of joining our ancestral lineages of body and mind.

I thank my daughters, Elena and Leia, for teaching me about love and human development. And my husband, Larry, for stoking the fire of love which has fueled the whole shebang.

Contents

Introduction

THIS BOOK CELEBRATES THE LIFE OF THE BODY—

ALL THE MYSTERIES, INTENSITIES, AND POTEN-

TIALITIES THAT HUMAN BODILY LIFE OFFERS.

❀ ❀ ❀

Why is there need to address such a basic aspect of our existence? Because, we have lost our connection to our bodies. Centuries of denial have reduced our experience of body to a mechanical one. The body in all its richness and sensuality has been driven out of town. As children, we learned that we shouldn't smell it and we shouldn't hear it. We were told that feeling it too much would lead to indulgence and distraction at best, or homicide and sexual mania at worst. We learned to view our body as an inarticulate machine that we should spend as little time as possible maintaining. And we were taught to keep it as still as possible. These are the denials of body with which we have been unconsciously indoctrinated. These deep denials in turn flatten our physical experience—an effect that further strengthens a mechanical view of the body.

My intention in writing is to reawaken within us the memory of our bodies' natural intelligence. By **natural intelligence,** I mean the synergistic intelligence that arises out of including all the resources of every tissue and fluid in the body. Every system of the body has its own unique abilities to perceive and respond. For both cultural and evolutionary reasons, we ignore and override both sensory input and behavioral responses that arise outside the nervous system. Including and integrating the intelligence and creativity of the entire body is natural intelligence.

As a somatic psychotherapist and director of the master's program in somatic psychology at the Naropa Institute, I explore human bodily life every day. The more I discover about the body's wisdom, the more I learn about human emotions, spirituality, communication, relationships, and politics. Often I find that studying the body reveals unexpected truths. I write this book to encourage all people to invite the body's wisdom into emotional healing, spiritual development, and our evolution as a global community.

In my professional development I have ping-ponged back and forth between so-called mind practices and so-called body practices. I have been a counselor, dancer, psychological researcher, bodyworker, Body-Mind Centering practitioner, and dance/movement therapist. The work that I have developed out of this journey, **body-mind psychotherapy,** integrates a deep experience of emotional and physical process down to a physiological level.

The field of **somatic psychology** centers psychological exploration in the body. This field originated in the 1930s as Wilhelm Reich, a psychoanalyst and close student of Freud's, moved beyond Freudian analysis to examine the role of energy flow and physical defenses (body armoring) in psychological health. Since then, a vast array of somatic psychological approaches have developed including bioenergetics, core energetics, dance/movement therapy, biosynthesis, hakomi, integrative body psychotherapy, and many more. Throughout the 1990s, practitioners of these different techniques have begun to create a unified field. Simultaneously, many traditional psychologists are recognizing the importance of including the body in their therapeutic work.

Studying the biological sciences deepens our understanding of human psychology. Within the history of somatic psychology, there is a rich tradition of incorporating research involving the natural sciences. Wilhelm Reich observed dragonflies, amoebas, and jellyfish; the application of his observations to the human psyche is still relevant today. Stanley Keleman, director of the Center for Energetic Studies in Berkeley, California, studies magnetic resonance images (MRIs) of brains and viscera in his quest to learn about how people shape their inner emotional worlds. Peter Levine, author of *Waking the Tiger,* observes animals in the wild to explore unrepressed response to trauma, applying those insights to the healing of shock and trauma in humans. Pre- and perinatal psychology investigates the impact of our experiences in utero and during birth on our psychology.

Other fields are also exploring the link between the natural sciences and psychology. Research in psychoneuroimmunology is revealing undeniable connections between the nervous system, our immune response, and our emotions. Behavioral medicine is attending to the personal and emotional factors involved in physical illness. Even general physicians are studying Eastern healing techniques that treat the body and mind as one.

My studies of motor development in infancy have led me to develop a basic template for human interaction with the world. I call this template **energetic development.** This is a process that relates our emotional maturity with the actual movements we use to move toward and away from the world. Energetic development explores the pathways of how we circulate our energy. This relates to **experiential anatomy,** which describes the qualities of energy along any given pathway. Experiential anatomy is an approach to the study of anatomy in which one seeks to experience personally in one's own body the aspects of anatomy that are being explored. My studies of experiential anatomy and physiology have allowed me to access the varying resources, emotional styles, perceptual perspectives, and the particular intelligence of the different tissues and fluids of our bodies. My studies of cellular life have revealed to me the potential for evolution and transformation that lies in the very core of our beings. Although much of my initial exposure to the physical aspects of these areas came from my training in Body-Mind Centering, to this work I have added a psychological perspective. This book shares what I have learned from both these perspectives.

In our rapidly changing world, the wisdom of the body has much to offer. We are seeking new solutions to our life on this planet. We are grappling with our next evolutionary step. We are reexamining our relationships to everything from spirituality to community, from pedagogy to global politics. Fundamentally, we are redefining human life on this earth.

These challenges and the solutions we seek are enriched when we inquire from the perspective of an enlivened body. By bringing the full scope of our intelligence to these issues, we will arrive at solutions that are livable. The cortical brain arrives at solutions that are possible, but the heart and guts must decide if solutions are humanly palatable. We have to honor both what we can imagine and what *feels* right. Our bodies hold the potency of all individual and communal exploration, supplying the juice, the breath, the concrete reality, and the resiliency that allow us to track and savor our development. How willing are we, really, to dive into the mysteries, the intensities, and the potentialities of our bodily lives as human beings?

This essential question leads to many important offshoots: Are we willing and able to be human animals with brilliant intellects? To feel in our bodies the inseparability of sexuality and spirituality? To experience the continuity of sensation connecting individual needs and group needs? To reacquaint ourselves with the community within our own bodies in order to practice community with others? Fundamentally, we must ask: How fully are we willing to look into our bodily experience for insights related to the mind, emotions, and spirit? Are we willing to let our bodies teach us, to integrate our natural intelligence?

A student approached me after class, saying, "I feel so frustrated with my learning. I watch you and I imagine that you are feeling all sorts of energy pulsing through you all the time, and that you are aware of all the different qualities and nuances of this energy." I asked her whether, in fact, this was *her* experience, *her* imagining. And she acknowledged that, yes, she had envisioned *for herself* this experience of fully living in her body.

Recently I saw a television program about the South American rain forests. A sixty-year-old man had shot a monkey with a poisoned arrow; the monkey was slumped fifty feet up a tree. The man was wearing a tiny loincloth, rendering visible nearly his entire body. The man grasped the tree with both hands and feet, his feet as fully engaged as his hands. With each reach he extended the full length of his body, then pulled his feet up just below his hands. Reach, pull, reach, pull, . . . in a moment he was up and then just as effortlessly down the tree with the monkey in tow. This was a normal event in the life of this sixty-year-old man.

Imagine if we joined this same tremendous physical aliveness, which is our birthright, with the visions and insights of our culture. What would human existence be like then? What, we must ask, is the potential natural intelligence of human beings?

This is the question I pursue in the writing of this book.

A practical note: In this book, I describe many personal experiences that illustrate different aspects of the material being presented. I have changed the particulars of each case study in order to protect the confidentiality of my clients, students, and trainees. Any names used are purely fictional.

CHAPTER 1

Concepts of Body-Mind Integration

The great gift of being in our world is the gift of the body.

—Stanley Keleman

ALL EXPERIENCE IS PHYSICAL. EVERYTHING WE DO—NOT ONLY OUR MOVEMENTS, BUT ALSO OUR SENSATIONS, THOUGHTS, AND FEELINGS—WE DO WITH OUR BODIES. OUR BODIES ARE INDEED A GIFT, BUT PERHAPS A GIFT WE HAVE SOMEWHAT UNDER-VALUED IN FAVOR OF OUR MINDS. TEACHERS OF ALL DIFFERENT PERSUASIONS REMIND US OF THE BODY'S IMPORTANCE IN THE BODY-MIND RELATION-SHIP. CANDACE PERT, A LEADING NEUROSCIEN-TIFIC RESEARCHER, ACKNOWLEDGES: " . . .YOUR MIND IS IN EVERY CELL OF YOUR BODY" (MOYERS, 1993). AND SUZUKI ROSHI, THE GREAT ZEN TEACHER OF THIS CENTURY, SAID: "BODY AND MIND ARE NOT TWO AND NOT ONE" (SUZUKI, 1970).

❀ ❀ ❀

Living in a Body

Hermit crabs borrow a discarded shell to live in. Caterpillars mutate in their cocoons and emerge as resplendent butterflies. As humans, our bodies are also changing shape and tone all the time. Do we envision them as discardable hulks or as transformative energy fields? How we think about our bodies is very important because it affects how we live in them. Do we feel present and connected within them or dissociated from them?

DISSOCIATION AND PRESENCE

Dissociation is a psychological term that describes a state of disconnection between one's body, one's feelings, and the present reality. This is a common experience of abused children and victims of violent crime and trauma: "During the incident, I felt like an observer—I wasn't really there." Even in everyday life, most of us are dissociated much of the time. "My mind was a thousand miles away," we say.

In contrast, **presence** is a term that implies connection. Think about the statement: "I felt it in every cell of my body." When all of our sensations, thoughts, and feelings are integrated, we are present in our bodies. The degree to which we are bodily present manifests itself concretely in each particular moment; in fact, being present in our bodies *means* being present in a particular moment.

We readily perceive bodily presence in others; we see it in their posture and movement, and we hear it in their voice and in the congruence between what their words and their bodies are saying. Overall, when a person is present in his or her body, there is simultaneously a quality of simplicity and vividness. Additionally, bodily presence often blossoms in an awareness of the body of the earth. Living more fully in our bodies can help us answer many of our questions regarding how to live responsibly with and on the earth. Considering these benefits, it's unfortunate that living fully in the body is so challenging for most of us. Let's take a look at why this is so.

INHIBITION AND CHOICE

To begin with, we can look at the powers of the human intellect. The earth cannot choose not to orbit the sun. An amoeba cannot stop itself from dividing. A wolf does not decide to hunt for prey. But humans have the power to inhibit our biological processes, our responses to our experiences, and our expressions of those responses. We also have the power to imagine and to choose options far beyond our immediate experience. We can imagine utopia in an evening's revery. We can choose to fly to Morroco or to hike across the

Grand Canyon. We are constantly making choices between one option and another: should I finish this chapter, or get up and stretch?

Having choices is directly related to the nature of our nervous system. As sensory input travels upward through the nervous system, it can be responded to with increasingly varied options. Emergency input is sent directly to the spinal cord for processing. At the level of the spinal cord, we respond reflexively. The ratio of input to options for output could be seen as 1 to 1. In the lower brain, the ratio might be 1 to 50; in the midbrain, 1 to 100; and in the neocortex, the part of our brain that is most uniquely human, the ratio might be 1 to 1000.*

Let's take the example of a bare foot stepping on a hot coal. If that coal is hot enough, it will elicit a reflexive response. We will quickly withdraw our whole foot. In this case, the sensory input went to the spinal cord and an immediate choiceless response was elicited, a 1 to 1 ratio. One input led to one response; there were no choices. If the coal was a little less hot, we might shift our weight onto that foot before the heat registers. In this case, the sensory input must go into higher parts of the nervous system to coordinate a motor response of shifting our weight and then withdrawing our foot. This would involve many options on several different levels. Finally, at the extreme end of the spectrum, imagine training in the yogic discipline of entering a trance state and walking on hot coals. In this case, walking on the coals elicits a rich array of spiritual visions, unique to each trial and to our level of attainment. At this level, the sensory input of the hot coals can result in a seemingly infinite possibility of neurological responses—1 to ?. We've gone through the ceiling of our previous ratios.

The point here is that it is human nature to be faced with multiple choices. A simple hierarchy in choice-making often leads us to pick one impulse and repress another. For example, I am laughing loudly. I see my neighbors over the fence. I quiet (or repress) my laughing so as not to disturb them. Our ability to inhibit biological processes on the one hand brings us seemingly infinite choices, creative richness, and civilized refinements, while on the other it brings disease, numbness, and perversity. Our choice-filled intellect is part of our biological inheritance. Optimizing the balance between choice and inhibition is a basic dilemma of the human body-mind.

EVOLUTION OF BODY-MIND DUALISM

What is **body-mind dualism**? How did it happen? If we examine the natural world, we see integration and wholeness. Trees, clouds, animals in the wild—all of these phenomenon manifest a total integrity. Where there are two im-

---

*This is oversimplified to illustrate a principle.

pulses, both are integrated. We do not find conflicting impulses anywhere in nature, except the human being. Somehow we have developed body-mind dualism, the ability to repress and ignore parts of ourselves which often results in opposing factions within our beings.

Let's retrace the evolution of body-mind dualism. Where did it begin? Four and a half million years ago with the human genus? Ninety thousand years ago with the human species? With the advent of agriculture in which humans began to manipulate nature? In the 1700s with the Industrial Revolution? Although we can never answer this question conclusively, examining related dynamics can deepen our understanding of it. To explore these, one must examine one's assumption as to the basic nature of body-mind dualism.

There are two different ways to approach this question. One view, which is an overly simplistic explanation, is that we have fallen from grace. The idea here is that we used to be integrated into the fabric of nature. We were children of the universe and, at some point, we somehow became split off. This is very much in keeping with the biblical story of Genesis. Eve ate of the fruit of knowledge and the human race was banned from the garden of Eden. We are left feeling that we made a big mistake and must go backward to solve it.

Alternatively, we could take an evolutionary approach. I find this premise much more rewarding. Perhaps it is quite natural that the unique capabilities of our species have led us to explore a lifestyle in which the mind dominates and ignores the body. It may be an evolutionary process to go through this phase of disintegration and reemerge into a new period of greater integration. Perhaps, by setting the body aside, we have been able to develop the full potential of our nervous system. Yet, in the last two hundred years, we have seen that our sophistication in science, technology, industry, communication, and transportation have not spared us from physical and psychological disease and the deterioration of our environment. Perhaps now that we are both confident of our intellectual abilities and cognizant of their limitations, we can enter a new phase of evolution, moving toward a reintegration of body and mind. Now that we have taken our natural intelligence apart, it may be time to put it back together.

Obviously, only a superhuman perspective could definitively affirm either of these theories as to the nature of body-mind dualism. My preference is to assume that we are evolving rather than falling. Maybe there's a bit of both going on. Whatever perspective one takes it is worth examining the religious and cultural dynamics that have accompanied the development of this split.

RELIGIOUS FACTORS

Indigenous cultures around the world share fairly consistent spiritual beliefs that see all life as connected to spirit and embedded in nature. Each species, including humans, is seen to have its unique but interconnected role. Similarly, the body and mind are inextricably connected. Joseph Campbell said, "The ancient myths were designed to harmonize the mind and the body. The mind can ramble off in strange ways and want things that the body does not want. The myths and rites were means of putting the mind in accord with the body and the way of life in accord with the way that nature dictates" (1988, p. 70).

This function of "putting the mind in accord with the body" is present in the teachings of Buddhism. Twenty-five hundred years ago, the Buddha recognized that the root of all suffering is the mind's struggle with reality, its rebellion against what is. This desynchronization between the mind and one's physical, embodied experience was seen as the very definition of suffering. Both Buddhism and Hinduism stress that all the gods and demons, all the heavens and hells, are within us. The great Hindu teacher Baba Muktananda was fond of reminding his students, "God dwells within you as you"—as the bodymind unity that you are. This view clearly supports body-mind holism.

The Western religions were born to some extent out of a revolt against the holistic beliefs of Eastern and primitive cultures. For long periods in the history of Judaism, Christianity, and Islam, clerics denounced indigenous worship of nature-based deities and promoted belief in a God who consists solely of spirit and is separate from and superior to lowly, embodied human beings. All three of these religions have teachings that promote denunciation of the body. The Old Testament, for example, teaches that the body is a vehicle of sin that must be purified and transcended. Women's bodies, which shed blood monthly and represent sexual temptation to men, are said to be particularly sinful. Thus, the earth, the body, and women all move into a place of denigration. In the fixation on heaven, the afterlife, and an external savior, there is a movement away from "putting the mind in accord with the body." The emphasis is shifted toward preparing for a heavenly afterlife.

CULTURAL FACTORS

Although it is difficult to separate religion from culture, there are some cultural factors that must be noted in the history of body-mind dualism. In *The Chalice and the Blade*, Riane Eisler (1987) documents the campaigns of warring peoples which dominated earth-based, goddess-worshiping agricultural peoples. An anthropologist, Eisler postulates that these campaigns to win new territories by force prompted a shift toward patriarchal culture that devalued both women and body.

Another important cultural shift occurs in the Golden Age of Greece. Here, the elevation of the intellect, reasoning, the art of debate, and the pursuit of science led to a confused interpretation of the relationship between nature and humans. For example, the myth of the young boy of Iassos tells of a boy who falls in love with a dolphin. He swims naked on his back daily with greater and greater sensual abandon, only to one day impale himself on the dolphin's fin (McIntyre, 1974). Also during this period, the Greek gods and goddesses came to be seen as more separated from earthly life, and the concept of Platonic perfection—the idea that the heavens contain perfect "forms" of which every object and creature on earth are only flawed imitations—was born.

Julian Jaynes (1976) postulates that an important development in the function of the human brain occurred around 700 B.C. While studying the works of the ancient Greek poet Homer, he noticed a change in the poet's writing between the earlier work, the *Iliad*, to the later work, the *Odyssey*. He noticed that in the *Iliad* there are no real uses of the first person singular ("I"), nor any real references to either the mind or the body. *Noos*, the ancient Greek word that comes to mean mind, is only used to refer to one's sphere of perception, as in "Zeus holds Odysseus in his *noos*." In other words, Zeus is keeping an eye on him. Likewise, *soma*, body, is only used in the plural, as when describing dead bodies lying around the battlefield. In contrast, the writing in the *Odyssey* produced decades later, reveals a highly developed sense of the self and a more specific definition and use of both the words *noos* and *soma*. Jaynes attributes this difference to a functional change in the brain, which has become fully aware of itself and able to self-observe. This, Jaynes asserts, marks the birth of self-consciousness. He notes similar changes within roughly the same time period in both the Mesopotamian and ancient Hebrew cultures.

It is also worth speculating about the effect of the development of written language which occurred around this time period. How did the ability to record speech affect our experience of the body, if suddenly a mind could be contacted without a living body present to represent it?

In the first centuries A.D., donations of land and money from wealthy rulers and simple peasants helped the Catholic church become increasingly powerful. Thus, its doctrine relegating the body to a lesser position and postponing happiness to the afterlife spread throughout Eastern and Western Europe. Women were denied positions of authority, and nature worship was punished harshly. By the Middle Ages, Christian asceticism—which promoted depriving and torturing the body to atone for sins—flourished. Enjoyment of sexuality and other physical pleasures came to be seen as sinful. All of these factors began to crystallize the body-mind split.

During the Renaissance, fueled in part by the rediscovery of classical texts and art, philosophers, scientists, artists, and rulers began to rebel against the limits imposed by the Catholic church. Several philosophical disciplines, which supported body-mind holism, developed during this period. For example, humanism promoted an appreciation for human values and embodied existence. Pantheism, the idea that God is everywhere and in all things, also developed during this period. These gentle philosophies may have supported the development of a more body-friendly culture if they had not been quickly over-shadowed by other, more dominant movements that emphasized the body-mind split during the 17th and 18th centuries: namely, rationalism, empiricism, materialism, mechanism, and reductionism.

Rationalism proposed that we can determine the nature of reality through the use of reason alone: experience and observation are unnecessary for knowledge. Its leading proponent, Rene Descartes, stressed the ability to think as the defining characteristic of humanity. Descartes' powerful statement, "I think, therefore I am," has reverberated through the centuries and continues to influence our culture today.

Also during the 17th century, the swift development of the natural sciences supported philosophies diametrically opposed to rationalism. These included empiricism, materialism, and mechanism. Empiricists investigated and valued only evidence derived from their sensory experience, ignoring anything they could not see, hear, smell, taste, or touch. Empiricism was accompanied by materialism, which held that matter is the only fundamental substance, and that spirit and mind—if they exist at all—are manifestations of matter. An outgrowth of these schools, mechanism came to view all living organisms, including human beings, as complex machines. Thus, empiricism, materialism, and mechanism together divorced nature from any spiritual intelligence, and further deepened the gap between body and mind.

As the 18th century progressed, scientists became increasingly confident of their ability to intervene in the flow of nature. Obviously, power over nature easily translated into inhibition of the body: self-control to the point of self-repression. This new attitude marked the beginning of a reductionistic tendency in natural science, an attempt to reduce life to its most basic mechanisms. The reductionistic approach has reigned in biology for centuries, and has led biological study away from any larger pursuits, such as understanding the nature of life or the synergistic magic of a living organism.

As science evolved, so did technology. Advances in production methods in the 18th and 19th century led to the Industrial Revolution, which extended the reign of the mind through machines. During the Industrial Age, mass production came to be valued over individual initiative. To harness workers to dangerous machines in dimly lit factories for 10–12 hours a day, individual bodily impulses had to be suppressed.

Accompanying the Industrial Age, Victorianism promoted a rigid sense of propriety over the so-called animal impulses. The result was an equation of human sexuality and other bodily impulses with immorality. For example, women who acknowledged their sexual urges were diagnosed by their physicians as mentally ill. Children were taught that masturbation was evil and even harmful. Homosexuality was punishable by death. Even Victorian clothing restricted and concealed the body: women's dresses—worn over boned corsets—had long sleeves and high necklines, and men's slender jackets, vests, and cravats were only slightly less restrictive. It is during this period that Western culture became thoroughly entranced in repulsion toward the sights, sounds, and smells of human physiology.

Although this somewhat superficial sketch of the history of body-mind dualism makes no attempt to illuminate cause, it does chronicle some of the dynamics that arose on the path that we as a species have been following for the last several millennia.

PRICE OF BODY-MIND DUALISM

We pay a high price for body-mind dualism. Our emotional and physical health is suffering. Recognizing our increased need for comfort, we have become increasingly grasping, consuming more material goods, watching more television, taking more medications, succumbing to addictions to gambling, food, shopping, alcohol, and other drugs.

Ecopsychology documents the ways that humans suffer from our divorce from nature and from witnessing the destruction we wreak on the planet. Feminism notes the ways in which our hatred of women limits our cultural creativity and leads to abuse of children. Our spiritual alienation, the breakdown of the family, all of these phenomena relate to body-mind dualism in some way. We see this litany of distress climaxing daily through global media.

On the other hand, we are making gestures in the direction of life, reaching toward nature, spirituality, community, and the body. The large-scale cultural gestures we are making toward the body come in forms like aerobics, health foods, and comfortable fashions. Although these may be somewhat superficial, they are nevertheless part of a cultural movement to reinclude the body in our lives. The question we must address is: how fully do we want to live in our bodies?

The Six Principles of Body-Mind Integration

If we are really going to integrate the body, we must do so in a way that acknowledges the intelligence and individual motivation of each part. The body is not a mindless machine that must be maintained or fixed. This is an antiquated view. Bodies are alive. They have their own internal motivation. This is true on every level—organismic, systemic, and cellular. All of our physiological activity has its own motivational integrity, its own emotional tone.

Wherever there is mind or intelligence, there is a sense of "what I want" and "what I do not want." This is a fundamental level of motivation. Motivation is the primitive root of emotion. In every minute physiological shift in the body, there is a quality of subjective individuality. Every sensation has some sort of emotional tone. We are alive down to a minute level. Even on a molecular level, life is naturally self-organizing (Kaufman, 1995).

Throughout the remainder of this chapter, we will explore six basic principles that I have found to be crucial to supporting the full creative potential in body-mind integration (see Box below). The rest of the book describes the practical application of these principles in the living body.

RESPECT

The first principle of body-mind integration is **respect.** Respect is an appreciation for the intelligence of the bodymind, its motivations, emotional tone, and responses. The body must be approached with respect for its intelligence and individual motivation. Whatever part of us we are addressing, we must respect the subjective, and even at times mysterious, nature of our bodily selves. We cannot fix our bodies as we fix a chair. We must ask our bodies, "How has the condition developed? What is the intelligent, healthy aspect of this pattern? What is the basic motivation here? Is there willingness to re-

---

SIX PRINCIPLES OF BODY-MIND INTEGRATION

Respect: appreciation for the intelligence of the bodymind, its motivations, emotional tone, and responses.

Full Participation: empowerment of each aspect of the bodymind to shift in and out of initiatory and supportive roles as appropriate.

Inclusivity: cultivating participation by all parts and aspects of the bodymind.

Dialogue: cooperative communication between parts and aspects of the bodymind.

Sequencing: uninhibited flow of energy within all parts and aspects of the bodymind and between ourselves and the environment.

Development: responsive, adaptive, and learning approach to living.

examine this strategy?" Rather than telling our bodies what to do, how to be we could inquire in a respectful manner. Like human beings, bodies do not respond well to being bossed around.

The second principle follows out of this. It is **full participation.** Full participation is the empowerment of each aspect of the bodymind to shift in and out of initiatory and supportive roles as appropriate. Often when we consciously approach our bodies or a part of our body for the first time, we seek to be aware *of* it. Full participation requires striving toward being aware *with* the body, not *of* the body. When we cultivate awareness *of* the body, we maintain a subtle distancing and objectifying of ourselves.

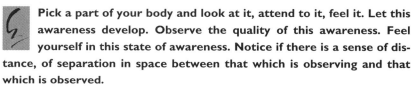

> **Pick a part of your body and look at it, attend to it, feel it. Let this awareness develop. Observe the quality of this awareness. Feel yourself in this state of awareness. Notice if there is a sense of distance, of separation in space between that which is observing and that which is observed.**
>
> **Now shift your attention *into* that part. Imagine that this is the part of you that sees and hears. Feel that this part is the very center of you. Again notice the subtle shifts in the quality of your sensation.**

Cultivating awareness *with* the body is a long-term and multifaceted practice. This practice, though subtle, is very important in that it invites the creativity of expanded resources. As long as we are merely aware *of* a part of our selves, it is not empowered to fully participate in a creative fashion.

Imagine, for example, the powerful ruler of a village observing from afar a young child in the village. The ruler notices the openness and sweetness of this child and wonders about the child's potential contribution to the village. The villagers are struggling with a problem, one that is complicated and difficult to overcome. They struggle and struggle and no solution is found. The child goes about his day-to-day business until one day the ruler stops the child and asks her about the problem. What would she do if she were the ruler of this village? As the story goes, the child's answer provides a simple and fresh solution to the problem.

This story exemplifies the possibility of full participation. What if we issue a blanket invitation that any part of our bodies can step into a leadership role at any time?

In many corporations today, there is a movement toward team work. As a culture we are realizing that the model of the silent mass of workers is not optimally effective. We are beginning to recognize that we need the creative input of everyone involved in a task to complete it well. By creating teams, we are potentially broadening our base of intelligence. This approach sounds good, and as those who have been involved in such a process know, it is an extremely difficult and evasive shift to make. Moving a group of people or a person or a part of a person out of a disenfranchised role and into a role of creative power and responsibility requires tremendous willingness to transform. Moving toward full participation is a process. And this is true on a bodily level as well.

Different kinds of resources are found in different aspects of our bodies. While our nervous systems know a great deal about discriminating, our blood knows more about nurturing flow. And while each of our basic tissue and fluid types have their own unique qualities and creative resources, on a cellular level we have a basic intelligence that is universal. It is our own nature, our human birthright to integrate and fully utilize all of these different levels and types of intelligence. Nevertheless, it is not an easy thing to accomplish; it is something we must learn how to do.

I wonder how many cultures, if any, have really mastered this integration of natural intelligence. It requires a body-based populace that listens to and respects the varied messages of all parts of the body. Which cultures, if any, have integrated fully developed intellectual creativity into a body-based approach? Which cultures, if any, have tapped into the full breadth of our human potential? Many earth-based cultures seem to have fully integrated much of the body's wisdom; our modern Western culture seems to be functioning pretty close to full intellectual capacity. Are we in a position to bring these two together?

Perhaps we are unequipped to ever fully assess this mystery. Perhaps we can only pursue greater degrees of integration of our own bodies and minds and invite more and more of ourselves into full participation. True integration requires full participation of all parts, that any group member can step into a leadership role at any time, offering unique resources to the task at hand. Any individual part can at times lead and at times follow, each in its own way.

INCLUSIVITY

This brings us to the third principle of body-mind integration: **inclusivity.** Inclusivity is the cultivation of participation by all parts and aspects of the bodymind. For full integration of body and mind to occur, *all* aspects of the body and mind must be consciously included. With full participation, we invited all of the parts of ourselves that we were aware of to fully participate—to shift into their own agency. With inclusivity, we are asking the parts that are invisible to our consciousness to come forward.

This is a huge order. Several decades ago, when we were at the beginning of our study of the human brain, it was a popular contention that most people only use 10 percent of their brains. This was a way to acknowledge the brain's awesome potential and mystery. Likewise, we could acknowledge the potential and mystery of body-mind integration. Perhaps we've only tapped 10 percent of this potential. Perhaps when we say, "I'm listening," or "I care about you," or "I'm working on this," the reality is that only 10 percent of us is involved. While it is powerful to move toward 100 percent participation, my experience is that even 60 percent is awesome.*

Let's consider the approximately 75 trillion cells in our bodies to be 75 trillion individuals in our organization. There are 256 different types of cells that we can think of as 256 different subsidiaries. Depending on how you divide them, there are about ten to fifteen different major body systems. That's ten to fifteen different specialties. What percentage of this constituency is respected, included, and fully participating in your organism? If each of these cells, cell types, and major body systems were consciously participating in our lives, we *might* discover new creative resources. We might have a radically different experience of our lives. What does this mean practically? We will explore this question throughout this book, but for now let's look at a practical example. As I write, I feel a warm, summer breeze move over my skin. I feel the pressure of the chair against my thigh. I also feel my focus of concentration centered around my eyes and forehead. I feel an intense vibrating of passion and intent around my heart. Noticing all this, my breath shifts. As I exhale more fully, I feel a deep stirring through my limbs and pelvis. What happened? When I consciously included my awareness of my head and my heart, my breathing shifted, my fluid circulation shifted. There were subtle shifts in my musculoskeletal system, which shifted my posture. The effect was that my overall state of awareness changed.

Including more of us always shifts our perspective and our creative resources. If you feel stuck in your life, try checking in with your body. Notice what you are ignoring and consciously invite it. New solutions inevitably arise.

This occurs in body-mind psychotherapy all the time. William is a middle-aged man who has just separated from his verbally abusive wife. He begins a session with the statement, "I don't know if I've done the right thing or not . . . and I don't know how to find out." His posture is one in which his heart is very retracted, and he is looking up out of this position with a slightly lost gaze. Upon attending to his body, he finds the highest concentration of sensation around his heart. As he explores these feelings in his heart, he finds that the emotional tone is one of anger. As he stands and allows his whole body to wake

---

*Obviously, quantitative assessment is objectively impossible, but attempting it can keep us humble.

up and acknowledge his heart, he feels empowered and strong, no longer really angry. I ask if he knows anything more about how he feels about his separation. "Absolutely," he says. "Absolutely what?" I ask. "It is absolutely right." At this point it is important to revisit the state in which he felt lost and unsure. Can he integrate these states so that it is not a black-and-white experience? This integration involves dialoguing between the parts of him that were afraid to leave the security of the relationship, and his heart, which felt angry about trying to protect him from the abusive qualities of the relationship.

DIALOGUE

Dialogue is the fourth principle of body-mind integration. Dialogue is cooperative communication between parts and aspects of the bodymind. Integration requires dialogue. The first principle of respect underlies dialogue. It is difficult to dialogue without respect. If I assume that your position is inferior, I will not listen openly. Equally fundamental are the second and third principles of full participation and inclusivity. This whole process is similar to developing a political constituency; one invites participation and then enters into a dialogue. One has to go into the backwoods of one's body to invite the voices back there to share their opinions. Other disenfranchised voices speak in the form of symptoms. Neither the silent ones or the symptomatic ones are really able to communicate effectively.

Learning the art of dialogue is a delicate process; the next chapter will discuss this practice. In a recent workshop a participant told of an internal conflict. Upon inquiring in her body, she found longing to go forward in her chest. In her belly, she found fear. When she invited those two parts to dialogue, the back-and-forth of the conversation consisted of "I can't," "Yes, you can," "I can't," "Yes, you can." That is a persistent stalemate, not a dialogue. What was needed was a process of cultivating awareness and communication so that the two parts could really negotiate, educate, and support each other, as in this vein: Chest: "I'm really eager to do this." Belly: "But I want to be quiet and alone. I'm afraid of doing that." Chest: "What is this fear like? Is it old?" The dialogue revealed the history of the fear, eliciting empathy from the chest that recognized a pattern of ignoring the belly and its fear. There was regret about this. The two parts negotiated a solution that included pursuing both quiet and solitude as well as pursuing the project.

SEQUENCING

As one establishes a dialogue, the natural outcome is a flow of energy and communication between the parts that are dialoguing. This flow of energy between parts of ourselves can be actively invited. In all of our activities, we feel most complete and effective when what is inside can come out and when we are able to "digest" that which we have taken in from the outside. We feel a sense of well-being when there is flow in our bodies. We feel connected when there is flow between us and the surrounding world. This movement of energy through our bodies is the fifth principle of body-mind integration: **sequencing.** Sequencing is the uninhibited flow of energy within all parts and aspects of the bodymind and between ourselves and the environment. Sequencing acknowledges the importance of communication in the body.

Conscious sequencing is like traffic control, the monitoring and encouraging of a healthy flow of traffic both within the body, and in and out through the body and the surrounding world. This traffic flow includes all manner of physical activities: muscular movement, neurological changes, a flow of sensations, breath, and more. Sequencing will be explored in great detail in the chapter on energetic development (chapter 4). For now, the following session will help illustrate. This session, one that took place many years ago, was pivotal in helping me learn about some of the fine points of sequencing.

 Frannie was a very hesitant, anxious young woman in her thirties who began a movement therapy session by describing her feelings of frustration and powerlessness. As she discussed her feelings, she collapsed and constricted her chest. Her breath became shallow and the vitality went out of her voice. I observed that her posture was initiated by her heart contracting back into her body. As Frannie talked, she spontaneously reached around and poked at a place on her back directly behind her heart where the muscles had become tight, outwardly manifesting this pattern of contracting the heart. I asked about this spot and she said it always hurt and she often wished someone would push on it for her. I offered to do that. [I would no longer be so willing to engage with her through touch. The use of touch is very potent in a psychological context and may bring up issues of preverbal relationship. Contacting the body without touch can often be as effective and allows the client to monitor interpersonal boundaries and their personal process more independently.] She wanted a lot of pressure and became very energized, pushing back very vigorously against my pressure. Her head and arms hung down passively. After a while, it became apparent that Frannie could engage in this relationship endlessly without variation. Comments regarding her mother began to surface spontaneously as she pushed, and even more so after we stopped. "I hate my mother . . . I love to make her mad." She felt powerful in relationship to her mother only when she was resistant. As Frannie talked she was energetically continuing this loop from her heart out her back. Her back hurt more; she wanted more pressure. It seemed to be a self-perpetuating cycle; therefore, I was no longer willing to push. I suggested she focus more internally—rather than focusing on the pain in her back, to instead feel what was on the inside in that area. She noticed a lot of sensation in her heart

and began letting her heart area move spontaneously. As her internal movements became larger and involved her face and arms, I encouraged her to let her face and arms be moved by her heart. Out of this, she found a dragon-lady character. Roaring, she seemed to spew fire: she drew her clawlike hands up into the air. Unlike the incessant pushing, this expression built, climaxed, and died down, leaving her in a calm and empowered state. Frannie stood squarely on her feet and looked me in the eyes. This was in contrast to both the victimized state in which she had entered the session and the resistant state she had explored. I told her that it was impossible to release the energy she experienced in her heart out her back, that only by allowing it to move out her face and hands and into direct relationship with the world could she experience that energy in ways that don't involve resistance. Frannie acknowledged that this was, in fact, what was happening.

In the beginning of this session, we can observe the sequencing from Frannie's heart into her back muscles. After attending to her heart, there was more conscious sequencing from her heart out her arms and hands, as well as out her face. Stagnant energy and tension are both issues of sequencing. When our shoulders are tight, we do not need to "get rid of the tension." We need to learn to allow that energy to sequence where it wants to go. Learning to work with our own state through a conscious stewarding and sequencing of energy allows us to appreciate our current state without fearing we will get stuck there forever.

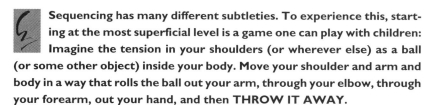 **Sequencing has many different subtleties. To experience this, starting at the most superficial level is a game one can play with children: Imagine the tension in your shoulders (or wherever else) as a ball (or some other object) inside your body. Move your shoulder and arm and body in a way that rolls the ball out your arm, through your elbow, through your forearm, out your hand, and then THROW IT AWAY.**

At a more subtle level, close your eyes and open your mouth. Feel the inhalation that happens involuntarily and the released quality of exhalation. Notice that in that exhalation there is a quality of allowing some energy that was stuck to move out through the body.

DEVELOPMENT

This appreciation of "where we are at" is easier when there is a trust in the movement of sequencing. As we learn to attend to the body and allow it to complete its own biological and emotional processes, we learn that we are naturally developing organisms. We change and we grow on our own. This is the sixth and final principle of body-mind integration: **development.** Development refers to a responsive, adaptive, and learning approach to living.

Somewhere in the puritanical underpinnings of the American work ethic lies a hidden belief that we are inherently slothful creatures and that we must use our wills to drive forward through that sloth. In the murky undertow of this belief, we blame our bodies for these slothful tendencies. Out of twenty years of experience in working psychologically with the body, I find this belief to be not only false, but backward. It is our estrangement from our bodies that leads us into sloth.

Earlier this year I took my computer in for a repair. The shop was in a windowless warehouse building. The repair person, who was overweight, lumbered up to the desk out of breath. While he was shelving my computer, two other employees came in and passed him without even a greeting. I was struck by the dehumanized quality of this workplace and asked him how he liked working there. He said it was all right, but that he was backlogged in his orders. He said that was frustrating and that he couldn't wait until the end of the day when he could go home and enjoy a glass of wine with his wife. I felt vividly struck by the barrenness of his work life. Imagining this, I felt saddened that this intelligent, communicative person was struggling to find compensation through food and drink in his evenings for the deadness of most of his day.

In working with clients, students, and myself, rather than finding sloth in the body I have discovered vitality living there. The body is movement. Within the body, we find the ceaseless, effortless activity of cells and molecules. Life is moving and fluid. By the most conservative estimate, the human body is 60 percent fluid. Our fluids are constantly flowing. Here is another source of constantly unfolding activity within the body. And all this movement is not just random and repetitive. Our bodies are responsive, adaptive, and learning. We are naturally developing.

Some organisms reach sexual maturity and then seem to plateau until death. Other organisms have the potential to evolve over the entirety of their lifespans. Biology has borrowed the term **neotony** from evolutionary theory to describe this. In neotonous creatures, certain qualities of infancy persist into adulthood. Humans are neotonous creatures (Montagu, 1989). Some of the crucial qualities of infancy that persist into human adulthood are play, learning, and development. However, in viewing our natural tendencies with suspicion, we have somewhat dampened our ongoing development. In our attempts to be "responsible" adults, we can limit play and stunt our development.

As we inquire into an emotional/physical experience following the previous five principles, there is always an opportunity for some sort of growth and learning, some sort of development. Approaching ourselves with respect, full participation, and inclusivity, we broaden our experience. Employing dialogue and sequencing, we invite development. In Chapter 4, energetic de-

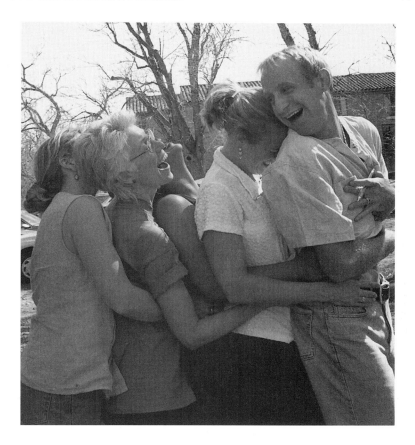

Adults at play.

velopment is discussed; to introduce the principle of development in body-mind integration here, let me share the following example from my own life.

A couple of years ago I began experiencing hormonal imbalances. My gynecologist felt that it was a part of normal aging process and prescribed hormonal and nutritional supplements for the rest of my life. I felt very discouraged. My image of myself in menopause was dry and gray. When I revived from my discouragement, I began an inquiry into the emotional and physical causes of this imbalance. Through meditation combined with emotional/physical processing, I evoked an image of my liver as an overworked and depleted frontier woman. Out of this, I began breathing into my liver whenever I felt any little twinges in its general area. This was several times a day. Almost immediately, my hormones became balanced. For a year and a half, my menstrual cycles were precisely regular. During this time I continued to breathe into my liver and I learned a great deal about my patterns of irritation and overwork. Actually, I did more than just learn *about* them. I am less inclined to overwork now and am more able to be active rather than become irritated.

After a year and a half, again my hormones became imbalanced. I felt extremely fatigued. I was distressed that the pattern had returned. Crying intensely about this, I felt an aching in the back of my uterus. Inquiring into the emotional tone of this sensation, I felt a subtle fear. Allowing this fear to sequence through my body, I quivered and jiggled. Completing this process, I felt tremendously energized. Now once again my hormones are in balance. Perhaps a year and a half from now, I will be better acquainted with my uterus. I might develop in related areas like sexuality and parenting. Who knows? Adult human development is not simple or predictable, but it is a reliable outcome of integrating body and mind. Furthermore, approaching life's process with a belief in development seems to invite further unfolding.

When we approach our process with an attitude of respect, we invite the full participation of all of ourselves (inclusivity). This broadens our range of experience. When we dialogue and allow sequencing, the process begins to move. By intentionally invoking development, often our lives unfold in surprising ways.

Personal Inquiry and Exploration

How has your personal history of body-mind dualism evolved?

- Physical influences include accidents, injury, over-medicalization of birth.

- Emotional influences include neglect, abuse, prolonged fear, lack of creative outlets.

- Educational influences include early stimulation of intellect, lack of creative stimulation, indoctrination in beliefs of body-mind dualism.

The six principles of body-mind dualism are **respect, full participation, inclusivity, dialogue, sequencing,** and **development.**

How have you learned to honor or violate each of these principles?

Note areas of your life in which you have experienced each principle at work.

Note a part of your body or an aspect of your life in which it might be beneficial to apply each principle.

Natural Movement

*Where does
movement come
from? It originates
in . . . a specific
inner impulse
having the quality
of sensation. This
impulse leaps
outward into space
so that movement
becomes visible as
physical action.*

—Mary Whitehouse

IN THE PREVIOUS CHAPTER, SIX PRINCIPLES OF BODY-MIND INTEGRATION WERE PRESENTED. IN THIS CHAPTER, **NATURAL MOVEMENT,** A PRACTICE THAT CULTIVATES THESE PRINCIPLES, WILL BE DESCRIBED. NATURAL MOVEMENT IS THE PHENOMENON OF SPONTANEOUSLY OCCURRING MOVEMENT THAT ALLOWS A NATURAL CONTINUITY BETWEEN SENSATION AND PERCEPTION AND RESPONSE, WHICH MAY INVOLVE MOVEMENT THAT IS LARGE AND VISIBLE OR MAY ONLY INVOLVE THE MICROMOVEMENT OF MINUTE SHIFTING IN THE JOINTS, OR INTERNAL PHYSIOLOGICAL MOVEMENT. NATURAL MOVEMENT ALSO REFERS TO THE PRACTICE OF ATTENDING TO SENSATIONS AND ALLOWING THOSE SENSATIONS TO MOVE, BREATHE, AND SOUND IN THEIR OWN WAY. TO INTRODUCE NATURAL MOVEMENT, LET'S LOOK AT AREAS IN WHICH NATURAL MOVEMENT SPONTANEOUSLY OCCURS.

❋　　❋　　❋

Natural Movement in Nature

Animals, children, and all the elements are constantly responding to the forces of life moving through them. Imagine a horse full of excitement—prancing, whinnying, rearing its head, tossing its mane. Of all the life forms on this planet only humans have the option of *not* responding with such immediacy to the forces of life. Through the twists of evolution, humans have the ability to shape, modify, and outwardly inhibit their organic responses to the world.

The British naturalist Charles Darwin (1809–1882) called the responses of animals **complete expressions.** Darwin believed that the full repertoire of animal movement that preceded us in evolution remains with us. For example, the complete expression of a person's sneer might appear as snarling and baring of the incisors.

Let's look at another example—a dog greets his human friend with a wagging tail. The dog's senses record the sight, sound, smell, and perhaps the touch of the human. The dog's cerebrum associates these sensations with pleasurable memories. This association is communicated to the endocrine system, creating a downward surge of excitement. The muscles of the dog's lower body are stimulated into wagging. The feeling of gladness and the wagging are continuous; there is a continuity of taking in and expressing out. This complete expression is spontaneous natural movement.

Bonnie Bainbridge Cohen (1993) talks about the infinite intelligent detail she perceives in the structure and activities of the sea squirt. This sedentary marine animal has a transparent, sac-shaped body with two siphons. When disturbed, it squirts water at the intruder. Thus, the creature's spontaneous natural movement enables it to circulate the ocean: the water goes in one end and out the other, both sea squirt and ocean being slightly altered and enriched by the process. When we humans respond to our worlds with our natural movement, we too are exchanging enrichment with our environment.

Natural Movement in Children

An infant is in constant movement, each movement a response to an internal sensation or external perception. Picture a newborn baby. Her senses receive the smells, softness, and contours of her mother's breast. She nuzzles into her mother's breast, in a complete expression of spontaneous natural movement. The perceptions coming in from the outside combine with a feeling of wantingness welling up from the inside. These perceptions and sensations sequence out as nuzzling.

Like the sea squirt, when the newborn takes in her mother's milk, the process of digesting it involves her whole body. She sucks the milk in and moves it through her body, scrunching and squirming—digestion made visible.

Or consider the toddler excited to see a friend. As they greet, he may resemble a horse we described earlier, prancing about, squealing in delighted anticipation, unable to contain his spontaneous natural movement. Unfortunately, by the end of toddlerhood, around age three, many children in our culture have already begun to inhibit their natural movement.

Expanding Our Concept of Movement

Movement is the circulation of innumerable forces through the vast array of different tissues and fluids of the human body. Outer forces that act on us include gravity, the quality and viscosity of the atmosphere, light, and the panoply of sights, sounds, smells, and personal and social events that we experience from moment to moment. The inner forces that act on us are the emotional and physiological responses to that which we take in. Usually we conceive of muscle and bone as the moving elements of the body, but with a closer look, we can see this view as myopic. All the elements of the body are alive and moving, though with very different rhythms and qualities. We perceive, process, and respond through all the elements of the body, which, like the sea squirt, act in concert to help us circulate our worlds.

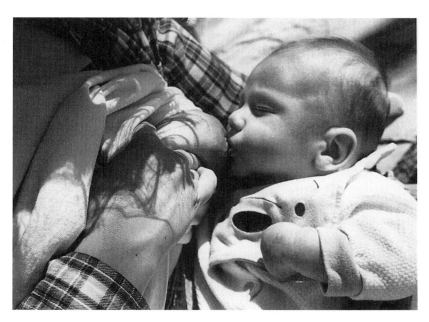

When the visceral organs respond, they move. The hollow organs of the body—the heart, stomach, spleen, pancreas, intestines, bladder, and uterus— are muscle, and like skeletal muscle, they move by shortening and lengthening, albeit in a more rhythmical fashion. The solid, fluid-filled organs of the body—the lungs, liver, gallbladder, kidneys, and gonads—shift position through changes in their shape and their connective tissue moorings.

Or consider cognition. Even our thoughts are molecular movements along nerve fibers between neurons in the brain. Sophisticated medical imaging devices such as PET scans show that thought occurs along certain pathways, making a shape in space and time.

On a muscular level, any thought also results in at least minute muscular responses, evidencing the body's compulsion to somehow *do* the thought.

Whether an internal process is a volley of dialogue within the endocrine system, a pattern of muscular response in the gut, or any other of the myriad internal physiological shifts through which we process that which we take in, it is movement, natural movement. We experience physiological processes as sensation, moving sensation. Sensation is inner physiological movement. When inner movement sequences out, it becomes movement through space, a visible expression of our state of being at that given moment in time. Imagine an adult working at a desk. She hears someone enter the room. That inner physiological movement of hearing sequences into a posture of looking to see what's been heard.

This inner physiological movement is not limited to sensation, however. When the phenomena that we take into our bodies are material in nature, we call the taking in *eating, drinking,* or *breathing.* When the phenomena are immaterial, we call the taking in *perceiving.* We process our food and drink, we are digesting. But the processing of perceptions—the play of the light or the emotional nuances of our companions, for example—though not as easily classified or named, is just as tangible, for it too involves a movement.

So whether a movement is as large and visible as a morning stretch, or as minute as perking up our ears, or microscopic as the movement of molecules through a membrane, there is continuity. Sensation, perception, and response continuously sequence from one to the next. Sensation is the movement of the sensory organs, which sequences to perception; movement of our neurons, which name and interpret the information and lead to a response, and again movement as we shift our relationship to our environment. There is the possibility of allowing each of these phenomena to move freely into the next—perception is movement that becomes internal physiological events that are sensation. Sensation is movement that becomes a response, a shifting of position or relationship to the environment. This natural continuity between sensation, perception, and response is natural movement.

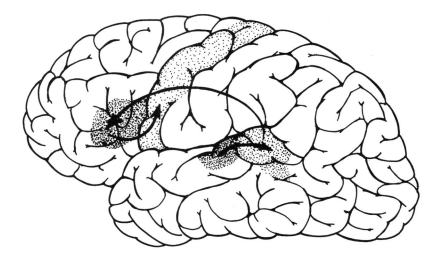

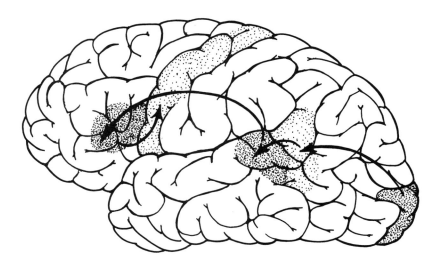

PET imaging of the movement of processing sensation and speech.

To experience the continuity of perception and sensation, pick out two of your favorite pieces of recorded music. Listen to the first closing your eyes and meditating on the sounds you are receiving. When it is over, notice how you feel in your body, observing particular sensations. Then, listen to the next piece in the same attentive way. Afterwards, when you check in with your body, are the sensations different from those with the first piece?

When we receive sensory information, we can perceive it more or less deeply. How deeply we perceive something depends, partially, on how open we are to allowing our responses to the perception to sequence through our bodies. Contrast the exercise above, in which you picked music you liked, to the experience of encountering a bad smell. Your face screws up in an effort to close your mouth and nostrils so that the smell can't get into your nose and mouth.

When we allow a continuous sequencing of sensations, perceptions, and responses to circulate through our bodies, we feel alive.

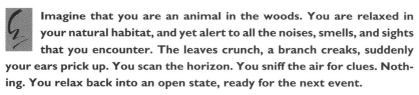 **Imagine that you are an animal in the woods. You are relaxed in your natural habitat, and yet alert to all the noises, smells, and sights that you encounter. The leaves crunch, a branch creaks, suddenly your ears prick up. You scan the horizon. You sniff the air for clues. Nothing. You relax back into an open state, ready for the next event.**

Like all mammals, we point our sense organs—our eyes, ears, nose, hands, and feet—toward or away from phenomena in the continual dance of perception, sensation, and movement. This is the natural movement of life. Imagine yourself a visitor in the ritual of a foreign culture. Feel yourself seeing, hearing, smelling, seeking to comprehend all the myriad information and to respond communicatively. Feel the small subtle orienting movements of your head, the delicacy of the breath that supports that, the balance of alertness and responsiveness that washes through your body as you take in, adapt, respond.

We are captivated by people who allow this continual flow of natural movement. We say they are graceful. We are drawn as to the Pied Piper.

On the other hand, most adults of our culture have learned to truncate movement—to stop it before its natural completion. We also truncate the flow between sensation, perception, and response, rather than let the movement complete itself seamlessly. Our brain recognizes where we are headed, and says, "Oh yes, turning the head to the right. I have a habitual formula for that."

 Pick an object in your peripheral vision and turn your head to look at it in your habitual way. Then come back to center. See the same object again with your peripheral vision. Allow your eyes to really

reach toward the object, drawing your head along as you go. Notice how differently you use your eye muscles and your neck.

Pick an object within your reach. Now reach for it and pick it up. Put it back in its place and return to center. See the object again. Wake up the skin of your hand by rubbing it. Imagine that you have never seen or touched such an object before. Let the skin of your hand reach toward that object, curious as to what it might be like to touch it. Notice the continuity of muscular activity from your hand through your shoulder. In the previous reach, it is likely that you predominantly used your shoulder muscles. What happened the second time?

Sensation is movement. We point our sense organs and grasp each phenomenon in particular ways. Perception is movement, which we experience as internal sensation. Our responses are movement. Sensation, perception, response: this is the continuous cycle of movement in which we live. The sequencing is not complete until we are brought into a new relationship to the environment, that is, until our internal expressions become externalized. Natural movement may be gross motor activity, micromovement in the joints or internal physiological activity. Engaging in natural movement can feel enlivening and refreshing. One of my clients recently told me it was like "taking a shower—inside."

Techniques for Natural Movement

Watching an amoeba moving through fluid, one can see the currents of water around it and the currents of the plasma within it. The membrane separating the two—amoeba from the water—responds to both but seems to maintain some intention as well. The membrane shapes itself to engulf a particle in the outer fluid. It does so without resisting or jumping ahead of either the inner or outer flow. We humans have infinitely more forces moving us at every moment, yet we can integrate this natural intelligence of the amoeba on many levels. Our membranes—in the largest sense the skin, nervous system, muscles, and bones—can shape themselves responsively to the internal flows of fluids, organs, and glands, blending that with intention. Conversely, we can ignore and suppress those flows. We can allow our membranes to be permeable, or we can rigidify. In movement, this spells the difference between *allowing* the body to move or mechanically forming it.

In natural movement, response is joined seamlessly to experience. If there is a crispness traveling out the nerves of your arm and your fingers are too numb to shape it, the energy is lost. If there is a lurch rising up through your guts but your neck is unwilling to let go of verticality, the energy is stopped in the throat. Able to control our impulses, many of us have lost touch with natural movement.

Natural movement is the manifestation of natural intelligence. To regain this intelligence we must actually practice our natural abilities. This is not an attempt to return to a simpler state. Rather, we can allow all of our natural intelligences, including cognitive thought, planning, and intention, to work together. Our uniquely human intelligence can be icing on the cake of all our animal abilities. The rest of the chapter describes four techniques for exploring natural movement (see Box below).

ATTENDING TO OUR SENSATIONS

The first step in practicing natural movement is attending very precisely to one's sensations. The language of the body is sensation. Sensations reveal to us the flow of energy in the body. We can therefore map the flow of energy through our bodies by charting our sensations. This process of mapping sensation in the body can be very helpful in developing bodily awareness. It is akin to charting traffic flow in a city. On a simple level, where there are a lot of sensations, there is a lot of energy. Where there are few sensations, there is less energy.

If you would like, take the time right now to attend to your sensations.

 Begin by standing or lying down. Letting go of your breath if you were holding it, begin to scan through your body for sensation. Let your body move a little and breathe to wake up sensation. Spend a few minutes just attending to all the sensations in your body as you move and breath. Let your attention move freely through your body from top

---

STEPS IN THE PRACTICE
OF NATURAL MOVEMENT

Attend to your sensations. Allow your attention to shift naturally from one sensation to the next.

Allow those sensations to move, breathe, and sound in an organic way.

Sequence sensations throughout your body, through your endpoints. Take time to wake up each endpoint by 1) really feeling the sensations in that endpoint; and 2) allowing those sensations to move, breathe, and sound in their own way.

Practice inclusivity to find the unexplored parts of your body.

to bottom, from outside to inside. **Notice areas that feel flowing or stagnant, dense or open, fast or slow. When you have gotten as much information as you want for right now, try actually drawing a map of your experience. This might allow you to sense even further.**

Allowing Sensations to Move, Breathe, and Sound

The next step in working with sensations is to allow each one to move,
breathe, and sound in its own way. This requires suspending ideas of what is
good for any one part of your body, and how that part should serve, acquiesce
to, or be dependent upon other parts. This is an aspect of the principle of respect. It requires moving your center of attention into the place of sensation
rather than viewing it from afar. To cultivate natural movement is to deliberately drop below your personal ideas of how you move, what kind of movement you like, what is beautiful, what is clever, what is aesthetically correct,

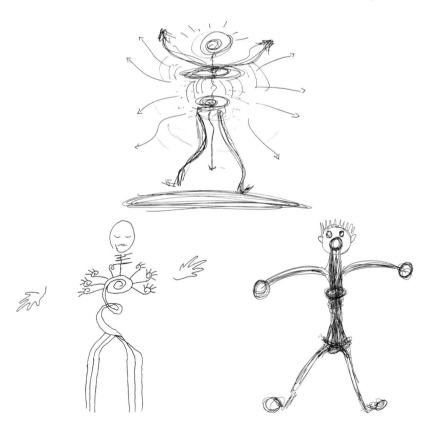

Energetic maps.

what is appropriate, and what is "good" for your body. Instead, attend to what you are experiencing right now.

 Let your focus be centered within whatever sensation comes to the forefront, and allow that sensation to move, breathe, and sound however it pleases (full participation). I often ask my students, "What if you had this body, with this energy, but no more rules about how you should move than a two year old?" For a short time, give attention and discriminating mind over to the body. Let it roam over its own terrain, not editing out the rocky slides or the peat bogs. Give the body an invitation to express without editing. Come back again and again to the basic perceptions of the present moment. . . . *I feel the skin tingling on the back of my neck. . . . I feel my right kidney making a fist.* . . . If you allow these feelings to move unobstructedly, how do they move? How do they breathe? How do they sound? Imagine that your sensation is a creature in and of itself. Let this creature invent its own activity.

SEQUENCING

The third practice of natural movement is sequencing, which we discussed briefly in Chapter 1 as a principle of body-mind integration. Sequencing entails following the pathways along which a sensation is moving and allowing the expression to continue until it has moved all the way through the body, that is, until it is fully processed. When information we have taken in is thoroughly processed, it becomes a response.

To work fully with sequencing, we must examine the basic layout of the human body. The major ports of the body through which information comes and goes are the **endpoints:** face, hands, pelvic floor, and feet. These are our primary contact points with the world. Our endpoints are the areas of the body in which our sense perceptions and motor abilities are most precise and detailed.

The endpoints are unique in several ways. Skeletally, the endpoints are composed of many small bones with multiple joints; they are the free ends of the skeleton. Many small muscles capable of precisely initiating and guiding movement compose the tissue of the endpoints. Neurologically the endpoints contain the highest concentration of sensory neurons in the body. All this suggests that the endpoints are in the best position to communicate with the outer world. They are important emissaries—major information passes through them. This is not to deny that every aspect of the body is continually receiving from and communicating with the outside world. However, the face, hands, pelvic floor, and feet are the endpoints of the primary pathways through the body.

The practice of natural movement involves sequencing movement in and out of these contact points, allowing them to shape the passage of whatever energies are moving through the body. In this way we support our energy coming into contact with the world.

 To experience this, feel your face. Take a moment to become aware of all the myriad sensations on the skin of your face, around your eyes, in your ears and nose and mouth. Begin to allow these sensations to move in their own way. Let your face contort and move. Also let it breathe and sound in any ways it wants to. As if it were its own little creature, let it invent its own movement and sound out its sensation. Try touching your face with your hands. When you are ready, reverse this. Let your face touch your hands, however it wants to. Do this until your face feels alive and fully present. As you move your face and allow your breath and voice to follow, how far down into your trunk can you feel this? How far into your trunk do the roots of your face go? Lay down and do this. Allow your face to move the rest of your body. When your face twists to one side, let that roll your body. Play with this as long as you like, but when you feel complete, notice how the energy is circulating in your body. Is it different from when you made your map earlier?

These same steps can be done with the other endpoints as well. Spending time attending to each endpoint fully can be quite luxurious. Why is this practice of natural movement simultaneously so energizing and recuperative? Because we are allowing individual free enterprise. This naturally releases vitality and flow.

The feeling of inner flow as well as the outer movement from the head down into the trunk is sequencing. Recognizing the continuity of perception, sensation, and movement enhances sequencing. Look up at the sky; feel the sensations of response in your body. Now look at a wall; how do your sensations shift? Perception results in sensation. When we recognize perception as sensation and sensation as a moving event, movement becomes a circulation of whatever forces are being experienced, within and without, from moment to moment to moment. Intentional sequencing invites this circulation. It primes the pump of flow.

PRACTICING INCLUSIVITY

The next step in the practice of natural movement involves inclusivity, which is, like sequencing, one of the six principles of body-mind integration. Our bodies are vast and varied landscapes. The trick in becoming fully present in the body is to find the unexplored territories. Within them there is sen-

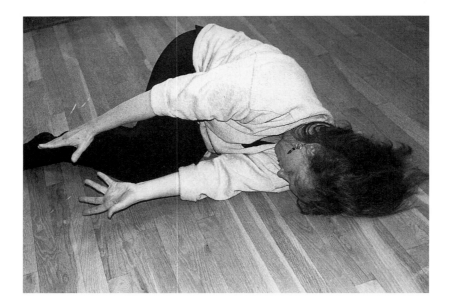

Waking up the endpoints in natural movement.

sory expression of all shapes, sizes, wavelengths, rhythms, colors, and textures continuously occurring. Culturally there are preferences to what of this inner experience we will attend to. There are also individual preferences. Aesthetically, we impose still more. As these preferences become fixed, we begin to lose our abilities to hear what we habitually ignore.

The challenge is becoming acquainted with more than the most familiar, most easily known parts, deliberately coming to know areas with more subtle voices. We have a tendency to come into unfamiliar territory in the body like a missionary, giving ourselves directives such as "Open up, release, soften . . ." Try coming in like a pilgrim, instead, asking, "What are your customs? How do you live here? What can you teach me?" This, again, is the principle of respect. With respect, one can really inquire as to how that part wants to move, breathe, and sound if given full permission. It might want to close, pull, grasp. It might want to hum or lurch. Maybe it wants to dissolve. All manner of rich and bizarre expressions can occur. Trusting this process to express some basic integrity is akin to trusting earthquakes, floods, and lightning as well as sun, rain, and blossoming.

Getting to know all of the body is quite a task. Parts of the body that have been ignored for a long time might need repeated attention before they respond. This is especially true if pain initiated the isolation. Pain is an important signal in the body. Its message is to call attention. Cheng Man Cheng,

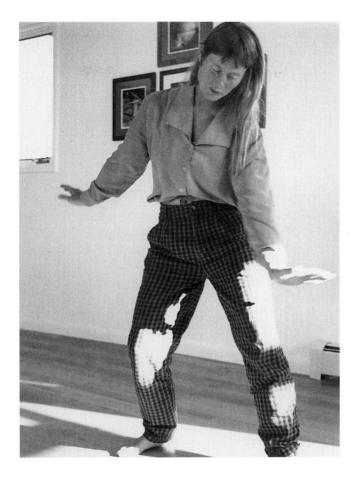

Sequencing in natural movement.

the famous tai chi master, is quoted as saying, "If you have a pain, rub it." This always makes me chuckle. It is so simple and direct, yet somehow, for our body-illiterate culture, it is profound. One of the terrible dangers of leprosy is the loss of pain receptors. In leprosy, a wound can go undetected and become infected. A leper vividly learns the value of pain. In our culture we are confused about pain. We try to camouflage physical pain with drugs. We try to distract ourselves from emotional pain. This is very different from attending to pain so that the emotional/physiological event can process and complete. An area that was ignored in pain can silently harbor that pain for years. When we ignore an area of the body, the circulation into that area decreases. We can slow our metabolism down locally so that a particular area can go into a sort of hi-

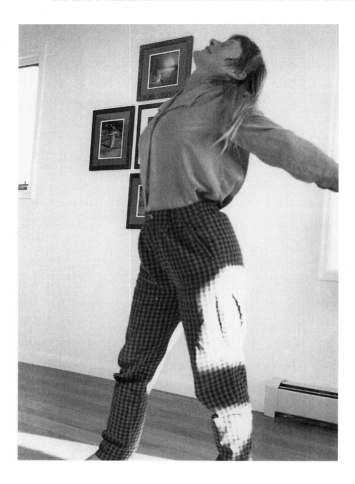

bernation or coma state; there is the minimal flow required to stay alive, but nothing beyond that. This is the opposite of full participation.

Dean, a businessman in his late 50s, had been adopted at birth and raised by an emotionally disturbed mother. He intelligently assessed his mother's confusion as a young teenager and left home as soon as he was able. From there he worked his way up in the music industry, becoming fairly successful. Beginning therapy was something of a novelty for him, a curiosity he pursued out of interest. Never married, he was intrigued by exploring his relationship to women. He saw a pattern of never opening up, never feeling wanted, never getting beyond a superficial level. When encouraged to feel his body and imagine some of the feelings that he might have experienced as an infant and a child, his sensation was predominantly in his heart. He cried and felt an ache in his heart. He said that he felt close to the therapist and realized that he had avoided closeness as a way to avoid feeling the pain in his heart dating back fifty years. As he revisited this process over a period of time, he simultaneously found himself experimenting with increasing intimacy with the women he dated.

There is a full spectrum of possibilities between coma and full participation. To invite areas that are withdrawn, one must cultivate an ability to attend to quiet sensations or numbness. Try the following exercise to practice inclusivity.

> **Ask areas of your body that feel painful or unfamiliar to speak to you. Inquire repeatedly if necessary: "Hello, anybody home? Well, maybe I'll just sit here and wait to see if anybody shows up. If you ever want to talk, I'm listening now. I know I've ignored you for years, but now I'm listening. . . . Well, I'll be back tomorrow." Make sure that you remain open to what is within the area.**

Imagine a child that has been hurt and ignored. If he slowly comes to trust someone's interest, opens up, and is then rejected or ignored, the child will close up even tighter. Often parts of our body react similarly. So you must be willing to tolerate the sensations that are flushed out. There may be intensity or there may be a gradually developing acquaintanceship. "Meet your pelvic floor. You haven't spoken in a while, but you were once good friends." "Here is your tongue. It knew you when you were a baby." "This shadowy figure you acknowledged in passing a thousand times is your liver, a magnificent storyteller." Even if the first sensations seem less than friendly, take the view that the more intensity there is, the more potential. Soon you might discover all sorts of wonderful indigenous expressions in your kidneys, throat, cerebellum, sacroiliac, arterial blood—expressions that are innate to the culture of that tissue, that fluid.

Another approach to expanding potential is noticing the sensations of numbness or stagnancy. These tend to be quiet sensations that may not draw our attention. We may not initially experience them as sensations. However, as one develops a strong relationship with louder sensations, we begin to notice that the quieter ones actually are sensations. They have their own distinct texture or quality. In working with sequencing you might stumble over areas that are somewhat numb or passive. Sometimes these areas might have developed their numbness out of neglect. Other times they might have been traumatized and never allowed to work through the trauma. Still other times they might have been instructed toward repression because they expressed an unwanted energy, such as anger, power, vulnerability, or sexuality. Whatever the case, it is possible to make a relationship with these sleeping or comatose tissue areas. Spend time inviting them and be open to any particular needs they might have. Once an area hears a sincere invitation and its particular needs have been met, it often does not take long to come into full participation. Spending a few minutes a day for two weeks is a sufficient amount of time. Don't be discouraged if it takes longer. Be creative about how you invite. Touch can help a great deal. The area may also have very complicated needs to fully participate. Keep working with reorganizing your life to include it. For example, if you are working with including your little toe, you may have to stop wearing shoes that pinch it. Or, if you are inviting your genitals you may have to totally revamp your relationship to sexuality. Whatever the case, to be fully alive all of our body must be fully responsive and expressive.

Benefits of Natural Movement

When we put our body through its paces, like a workhorse, all of these subtle impulses are ignored or actively repressed. By living only within the confines of habitual movement, these subtle impulses are harnessed, joined to some larger cause. In either case, the natural intelligence of the body is not being allowed to surface. When we enslave or make an object out of some part of the body, it loses touch with its own potentiality. Its mind becomes enslaved. Think of domesticated animals who lose their spirit or released prisoners who have to "learn" to be free. Often there is a cost for slavery that extends beyond its end. The body functions in the same way. Each part has a need to express itself. When it is continuously suppressed or constantly in a role of supporting the expression of other aspects, there is suffering. On the other hand, when someone moves the way they really feel, it is very pleasurable to watch. When I witness someone living in a body with many silent members, many parts of the body whose impulses are not being expressed, I want to say, "Wait, you forgot your feet," or "Excuse me, your intestines have been trying to get your attention." What we have learned not to feel may speak very loudly without our hearing it. The forces we have learned to ignore may actually push and pull us quite forcefully.

Through practicing this technique of natural movement, we discover our interior landscapes—all manner of wonderful shapes, densities, and rhythms to which we can attend. The attention of our living tissues and fluids will naturally sequence out into the space around us if they are so allowed. Body awareness does not mean being aware *of* your individual anatomical parts, but being aware *with* all of you—all of your muscles, your guts, your glands, your teeth, and your toes—all tuning forks through which you can hear the movement around you.

Natalie Goldberg (1986) says of writing, "You listen so deeply to the space around that it fills you, and when you write it pours out of you." So it is that when you really live, you listen deeply as space moves through you. *The hardness of the floor . . . I feel it first on the soles of my feet, then it echoes on the in-*

side of my knee. It's a cold surge in my belly. The whoosh of a hand past my face flutters in my heart. My skull longs to touch it.

Our perceptions naturally move us. As humans, we have to unlearn the inhibiting of our responsiveness. Similarly, we do not have to invent a relationship to space—we can allow it. Movement is the joining of inner and outer space.

Movement is natural when the forces that motivate it are not lost in the expression, when the movement is not stopped before its energy is spent, when the expression of one force supports rather than inhibits another, and when the relationship to space is enlivened and continuous. The practice of natural movement works to liberate responsiveness to energy as well as sensitivity to the choices of human intellect, seeking to cultivate the full range of intelligence—amoeba to wild horse, infant to adult—which is our heritage. Through the process of natural movement we can more fully embody ourselves, our life's process.

Personal Exploration

Practice finding sensations in your body and describing them verbally. Generate new words to describe each sensation. Expand your repertoire over time.

Practice finding particular sensations and embodying them with your whole body, i.e., if your head is throbbing, let your whole body pulse to that rhythm.

Practice finding sensations and allowing images to develop out of them.

Choose an easy, comfortable amount of time for a first experiment with natural movement. Ask yourself if you want to begin by standing, lying, or sitting. Begin by scanning your body for sensations. Based on that, get an overall sense of your energy flow. Begin letting your attention shift from sensation to sensation. Allow each sensation to move, breathe, and sound however it wants to. Continue for the predetermined amount of time. . . . Afterwards, notice how you feel. Compare that to how you felt when you began. Spend some time writing about any images, emotions, thoughts, or any other particular experiences that arose.

CHAPTER 3

Embodied Relationship

I'm in an eternal sea of continual pulsing patterns, and this is a bodying pattern. From the beginning of my existence, I am in something and it's pulsing me, bodying me. And it is bodied.

—Stanley Keleman

LIFE ONLY EXISTS IN RELATIONSHIP TO OTHER LIFE. WE ARE BORN FROM THE WEB OF LIFE TO INHABIT OUR BODIES WHICH ARE ALSO EMBEDDED IN THE WEB OF LIFE. WE ARE ALWAYS EMBODIED. WE ARE ALWAYS LIVING IN RELATIONSHIP. WE ALWAYS LIVE WITHIN A BODY WITHIN THE WEB OF LIFE. FROM THIS POINT OF VIEW, THE ENTIRE PHYSICAL WORLD SUPPORTS EACH INDIVIDUAL LIFE. BUT WE DON'T ALWAYS EXPERIENCE THIS, PERHAPS BECAUSE ANOTHER ASPECT OF HUMAN NATURE DRIVES US TO SEPARATE OURSELVES, TO TAKE OURSELVES APART. WE ARE TINKERERS. WE DIVORCE OURSELVES FROM OUR BODIES, THEN SEEK TO BECOME EMBODIED. LIKEWISE, WE CREATE AN ILLUSION OF ISOLATION WITHIN THIS WEB OF LIFE; OUT OF THIS, WE SEEK RELATIONSHIP. JUST AS WE ARE CONFUSED ABOUT THE RELATIONSHIP BETWEEN BODY AND MIND, WE ARE CONFUSED ABOUT THE BALANCE OF INDIVIDUALITY AND COMMUNITY.

❀   ❀   ❀

Perhaps, a further evolutionary challenge is involved in this issue. For the last few hundred years, the notion of individuality has been manifesting. Before that time, the tribe or feudality or church or nation was consistently the first priority. The individual yielded to the communal. In the last few hundred years, we have made individuality a priority. The creation and rise to power of the United States, a nation that exalts individual freedom, symbolizes this shift. The art of antiquity is impersonal: neither specific artist nor specific subjects are spotlighted. Only in the last few hundred years have we had the phenomenon of particular artists painting individual portraits of everyday people. We have come to value individuality; often this is at the expense of community. Perhaps we are now facing the evolutionary challenge to integrate individuality and community.

There is a parallel between the relationship of individuality and community and that of body and mind. Both relationships may either be integrated into a complex whole or polarized into an irreconcilable duality. As we seek to reconcile the relationship of individuality and community, we might be tempted to repress some of our internal impulses, further polarizing body and mind. These are complex issues that require a broad perspective; however, once again, I will advocate for the wisdom of natural intelligence as an avenue toward further evolution. By feeling our bodies and dialoguing, we can navigate a course that honors both our individual bodymind and our community.

This chapter begins by exploring the ways in which our body-mind duality can become further exacerbated in relationship and describes some techniques for working with these dilemmas. As we bring our bodies more directly and honestly into our relationships, the balance between individuality and community becomes both richly complex and ultimately integrated at a deeper level. The chapter ends with a discussion of the embodiment of the ultimate relationship, our relationship with spirit, our spirituality.

Socialization and Embodied Relationship

Our culture believes there is an inherent conflict between individual bodily impulses and social order. A somatic view offers a different perspective. By living *in* our bodies, being engaged and aware at the sensate level, we can feel both the sensations that arise from internal events and our responses to external events. We can also feel the way in which our internal and external sensations integrate to express a unified response, one that balances inner and outer needs without conflict. This is embodied relationship. Imagine this situation:

I am hungry. I sit with a hungry child. A small amount of food is placed between us. If I am attending only to my internal world, I will eat all the food. If I attend only to the hungry child, I will feed the child all the food. If I am attending to both my internal and external environments, I feel my own hunger pangs and the dullness in my limbs and eyes brought on by a low blood-sugar level. Sitting with this child, I see her hunger manifest as distress on her brow and in her shoulders. I smell and feel her state. I instinctively weigh our shared hunger, our shared need. I feel this measuring and reasoning in my body. As it mixes with my own sensations of hunger, I breathe deeper. I perceive more space around my eyes and my belly. The child and I eat slowly, sharing the food as we gauge our needs.

In this hypothetical situation, the child and I each sense our own needs at the same time as we sense the environment around us. Hearing, seeing, and otherwise sensing the external world are inherent physical functions that register deep in the body. Personal needs do not belong solely to the body. Universal needs do not deny the body. Communal impulses toward universal well-being can be found by resting deeply into the body.

As part of our socialization process, we have been taught to *not* feel these communal impulses. We have been conditioned to believe in a basic schism between our animal bodies and our human potential. The split between our animal intelligence and our human potential is well established and diligently maintained by our culture. The language we use polarizes the two. The belief deepens into a functional desynchronization of body and mind. Out of this desynchronization, we have the experience of rhythmical chaos, abandonment, deadening of energy, constant interruption of natural cycles. We see, hear, and feel other people living from an incredibly meager portion of their natural intelligence, their natural aliveness. These experiences reinforce our belief in the desynchronization of body and mind.

We first observe this schism in relationship. It results in a lack of meaningful communication. Repressing our bodily process renders relationship with others less satisfying and meaningful. We feel that the relationship is not working. In an attempt to solve relationship problems, we repress our bodily responses more. The whole process can snowball into a sense of being alienated from our bodily selves *and* from others. We learn to merge with others or isolate within ourselves. Either of these courses creates a feeling of alienation from ourselves and from other people.

From this perspective of alienation, we have formulated our view of human nature. As part of our socialization, we come to believe that human nature needs to be repressed, that human nature has innate difficulty integrating individual and communal impulses. Perhaps, from this limited view, we have underestimated ourselves. Recognizing our culture-borne biases about human nature and human interaction is extremely important as we work with integrating natural intelligence into our interactions.

We forget that we are animals. When we look at other animals we don't apply what we see to ourselves. We don't recognize that we could have as much energy as a galloping horse. When we observe two or more dogs meeting, we don't recognize our own abilities to be so direct. The truth is that we, as mammals, have the same basic faculties, capacities, and prowess shared by all mammals. And all mammals carry within all the potentials and abilities of previously evolved life forms. We could learn much about human nature and interaction by studying other mammals.

We don't even apply to ourselves the lessons that come to us from observing the behavior of children. We believe that only children should hop and skip, only babies should appear so in awe, so open and curious. We believe that it is childish to squirm and giggle and cry.

As children we learn very quickly where we are headed. We are headed toward adulthood, which is a very serious state devoid of many normal animal behaviors. Who is an adult? From the child's perspective, an adult is someone who doesn't laugh fully or very much. An adult is someone who doesn't cry or play or fight (openly). Adults don't move their bodies without specific purpose. And they don't make any nonfunctional noises. If they do so by accident, they utter an embarrassed "Excuse me" right away. An embodied definition of adulthood might include earlier repertoires. We are a shifting kaleidoscope of every age and every species that we have ever been.

The cultural body shrouds our animal bodies. By dictating how we move and breathe and speak and what we feel, the cultural body determines the totality of how we interact. Our interactions are in turn shaped by our societal norms pertaining to gender, age, economic level, race, and profession. These rules are all intricately relational, dependent on who is interacting with whom. For example, the cultural body encourages women to speak at a pitch toward the upper end of their register and men to speak at a pitch toward the lower end of their register. This becomes more noticeable when a woman is speaking to men than it is when she speaks to other women or children. The cultural body allows women to move their pelvises in certain ways, men in others. There are many gender differences defined by culture. These rules become more complex as they are dictated by particular relational hierarchies.

Economic and racial norms also dictate such physical parameters. Visiting my home state of Virginia, I noticed a major difference in the demeanor of many African Americans. When I was young, African Americans only showed their sparkling eyes and full chests in private gatherings. I was amazed to see some African American people now breathing fully out in public. I was grateful to be shown so directly that indeed the cultural body *is* mutable, and, in this case, moving toward more embodied interaction. As the cultural rules shift, relationships can change too.

Another form of cultural conditioning is implied in our attitudes toward health and healing, or to be consonant with the viewpoint of our culture, in our attitudes toward disease and medicine. From an early age most of us are taught that the quiet signals of distress that we receive from the body are incomprehensible and should be ignored until they get to the point of prolonged pain. At that point, we should take our body to the doctor so that the medical world can change our state for us, interrupting our bodily processes. This external prescription, symptomatic of our disembodied culture, conveys the message that we do not have the resources or instincts to support our own healing processes. This medicalizing and pathologizing of our animal rhythms begins with our most dramatically creative act of life—that of giving birth and being born. Birth is treated as a disease process that must be subdued and controlled.

The sum total of these many cultural influences is an injunction and agreement to subdue and deny bodily life, both within ourselves and within our relationships. As a culture we have come to view our bodies as tremendously limited. We cannot imagine running all day holding a single mouthful of water, as the Apaches did, or fasting to release energy as yogis do. In relationship we cannot imagine touching one another the way people of some "primitive" cultures touch one another, freely without inhibition or invasion.

This policy of controlling the body strongly influences our emotional lives as well. As part of our socialization process, we learn to conceptualize our emotions so much that we only vaguely remember that they might have something to do with the body. The labels we use to describe our feelings—words such as anger, joy, love, fear, sadness—have taken on meanings of their own. We forget that these are very general terms that approximate extremely specific bodily responses and sensations. Taught to ignore our bodily energetic states, we have been encouraged to invest heavily in the verbal currency that describes these states. The result is that we go so quickly from the bodily sensations to the verbal label that we forget *how* we know what we are feeling in the first place. *Emotions occur in the body.* How do we know we are angry, happy, fearful, or overwhelmed? Our bodily sensations tell us. When we lose contact with these sensations, it becomes very difficult to communicate emotionally with others. Talking about our feelings without involving our bodies can become an indecipherable mess.

This is another roadblock in embodied relationship. If we cannot talk about our personal experience clearly, we cannot share at an emotional level with others. To share emotionally with others, we need to be able to validate our own feelings, recognize the difference between a feeling and a thought, and recognize the difference between our own experience and that of another. Instead, our socialization process encourages us to remain unconscious of the feelings in our bodies. At some point the amalgam of sensations that constellates around an emotional experience registers in the conscious brain as a one-word label. While we are aware of the definition of that label, we often block out of consciousness the physical sensations on which the label is based. Ignoring our personal physical ground of emotions, we commonly validate them through claiming external cause: "I am happy because he loves me" or "I am angry because she is so irritating." Conversely, we invalidate feelings based on a lack of external cause: "What right do you have to be angry about that?" or "You don't have any reason to be sad." This is tremendously confusing in a relationship.

From a somatic point of view, *emotions are valid purely because they exist*. We can manipulate emotions by our attitudes toward them; however, we cannot wipe emotions out of existence. We can suppress our awareness of our emotions, but we cannot rid ourselves of the palette of sensations from which they arise. Even in the early years of psychotherapy, it was recognized that repressed emotion was often underlying conditions of hysteria and psychosomatic illness. The current attention to stress-related illness acknowledges the reality that suppressing emotions affects physical well-being. The word *emotion* comes from the Latin *exmovere*, meaning "to move out." With an accepting attitude toward emotions, our bodies instinctively allow the feelings to "move out," to sequence and release. However, this embodied attitude toward emotions has been all but lost in our culture. We have deadened the aliveness that is our evolutionary inheritance, the aliveness that is the gift of our natural intelligence.

Integrating natural intelligence into our interactions can be a risky and wild adventure. As we experiment with feeling our bodies, it may seem difficult to attend to others. We may find it challenging to skillfully express what we feel inside. We may discover parts of ourselves that we have ignored for so long that we don't know how to include them in our current lifestyle. With practice we become more creative about bridging our internal process with the outer aspects of our lives. There is no need to sacrifice one for the other. However, initially you will need to be open to experimentation to integrate inner and outer demands.

The hallmarks of embodied relationship seem to be honesty and directness, deep bodily satisfaction, and profound contact and exchange. As I live more fully in my body, I feel more civilized, more communal in my motivation. How paradoxical this is to the dogma of body-mind dualism, which teaches that listening too much to our bodily selves will result in selfish, irresponsible, immature, and potentially dangerous behavior.

In Chapter 1, we discussed the basic reality that, living in a body, we are by definition body-centered. We are self-centered. Culturally, we are taught that this is a bad thing; selflessness and self-sacrifice are the virtues to which we are taught to aspire. Theoretically, these virtues should create a society based on kindness and lack of attachment to personal gain. The unfortunate reality is that our cultural values appear to tend more toward competition and greed.

 I was privileged to sit next to a lovely woman during a plane ride. Her story illustrates the healing nature of discovering a positive sense of selfishness. She was Israeli, but was born in Poland. Very vital and animated in her speech and manner, her eyes were quite wide open and her irises were covered with the tiny dots that iridology calls stress marks. She told me of her life in Israel. Her children were grown, with successful professions and families. She had retired from her life-long work as a teacher and had created a very interesting regimen for herself. She awoke each morning and drank the juice of several lemons from her lemon trees (through a straw so as not to harm her teeth). She walked for an hour and while she walked she practiced a sort of body-mind meditation that she had invented. Then she came home and played piano for four hours. "I love it . . . maybe it is selfish, yes, well, I am selfish . . . . All my life I cared for others, now it is my turn." We discussed the philosophy of giving, using our plastic cups and melted ice cubes to illustrate. Is giving about emptying my cup into yours, or is it about letting my cup fill and overflow into yours? She told me of her early life in Poland. Her family had a large apartment with a beautiful grand piano. They were wealthy and artistic. Then she found herself in an orphanage in Israel. She remembers nothing in between, but was told that her entire family was killed and that a family friend somehow hid her away. I told her I felt very inspired by what she was doing with herself—that what she called selfish sounded very healing to me. Maybe she was allowing her cup to fill in a way that it never had.

How do we learn to be selfish, "self-centered," in a positive way? We must first question the benefit of assumed altruism. If my compassion or generosity is based on a concept that I don't feel in my body, how is that different from giving out of a body-based desire to give? When love, attention, or support feels pleasurable to give, it is much more pleasurable to receive. Obligatory responses feel hollow and only temporarily or partially satisfying. Furthermore, they may leave us feeling that we "owe" our benefactor. On the contrary, responding from our own impulses can be immensely satisfying.

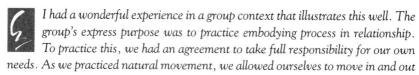 *I had a wonderful experience in a group context that illustrates this well. The group's express purpose was to practice embodying process in relationship. To practice this, we had an agreement to take full responsibility for our own needs. As we practiced natural movement, we allowed ourselves to move in and out*

of contact with each other as we felt our attention naturally shift. Each person was responsible for continually grounding in his or her own experience and communicating what he or she wanted and did not want from others. At one point most of the group was involved in individual activities. One person said, to no one in particular, "I want to hear everybody make a really loud noise." The rest of the group pretty much continued their previous activities. Nobody made any loud noise. One member said quietly, "I feel like being quiet now." The moment passed and was consciously forgotten, but about half an hour later, the group found itself engaged in some of the loudest group activity I have ever heard. Some people were singing, some were shouting. It all seemed to arise spontaneously out of the moment. Yet in discussing this later, everyone felt it was definitely, in part, a response to the previous request. There was a unanimous agreement that the experience was immensely satisfying for all concerned, so much more satisfying than an immediate, obligatory response would have been. If we do something we don't want to do, we miss the opportunity to do it when we do want to. Our deep indoctrination of mistrust for the body has confused our basic sense of generosity and compassion.

Our endpoints can also help us learn to embody our process more fully in relationship. When they are plugged into the world's sockets, we feel energized, available to give and receive. How much voltage can these connections carry? This may be a function of how available the endpoints are. Glazed eyes, listless hands, pursed lips, a slumped pelvis, tension and gripping in any of the endpoints—all of these can be signs of not being engaged with the world.

Practices in Embodying Relationship

My experience is that most of us are not practiced in being physically present and honest when we are in relationship to others. Being present in relationship is so contrary to our habitual rules of conduct that we need to practice, working in small increments. While the increments described here might initially sound very elementary, practicing them is powerful and challenging.

Before practicing embodied relationship, we must be aware of how our energy is circulating in our bodies. Using the practice of natural movement, we become as clear as possible about our personal experience in this moment. Also, it is important to really sink our attention into our bodies so that we keep coming back to our own experience as a ground. In the course of an interaction, our attention, when allowed, will naturally circulate in and out— through the body, out into the environment, and back through the body.

For most of us, feeling our own bodily experience and attending to others is so difficult that it seems impossible. In developing the material presented in this chapter, I taught a series of yearlong classes. For the first half of the year, we would work with embodying process with no interaction. When, in the second half of the year, we began to interact, people often found it difficult to stay fully in touch with themselves. The practice was to keep coming back to how the energy was circulating in your body and to use this as the guide for when and how to interact.

Habitually, however, we tend to act according to expectations rather than allowing this natural circulation of attention. This may cause us to get stuck either out or in. My attention may be so introverted that I am not able to make contact, or so extroverted that I am making empty contact. In this case, there may be lots of interaction with the world, but nobody's really home. There is the illusion of giving and receiving, but not a real exchange.

 Try this simple exercise with a friend. First ground yourself in your own process. Spend time breathing and moving with yourself. Map your energetic state following the directions in the previous chapter. In a standing position, breathe intentionally and sequence energy through your whole body. Check in with your endpoints. Are they all awake? Is there a free passage of energy in and out of them? Now move across from your friend. See if you can continue to stay awake to your own body. Let your eyes move in and out of contact while you observe your internal shifts in response to being with your friend.

Does this sound incredibly simple? Try it. It may surprise you. Does your overall level of awareness diminish? Do you habitually shut down in certain areas? It is a very difficult thing for most people of our culture to stay in touch simultaneously with their bodies and with another person. When speech is part of the interaction, we enter into the realm of an advanced art. The basic skill of embodying process is allowing contact with oneself at the same time as contacting another. How often do we shut down our awareness of our own experience when we are in contact with another person?

Human contact can be an elusive experience. We have all heard someone say, "I just didn't feel that he was really listening to me," or "I just didn't know how to reach her." Defining contact on a functional level can connect it more easily to a bodily experience. By isolating the concrete functions of contact, we have a way to practice and learn *how to be in contact with others*. Contact with another is only truly possible when one is in contact with oneself. On a concrete level, contact includes attention on a variety of functional levels: proximity, touch, eye contact, speaking, and listening.

Proximity refers to the distance between two people who are relating. When proximity is a fully embodied process, we see the distance between two people being sculpted and changed in a constant energetic dialogue. By

touch, I mean actual physical contact between any body parts. An embodied relationship to touch is satisfying to both people involved. It is neither invasive or demanding. **Eye contact** is also used here in a simple, practical way: the literal meeting of two people's gaze. So much is communicated through this subtle form of exchange. **Speech** is an activity that most of us do so often that we are very unaware of our manner of speaking. Embodied speech explores the possibility of speaking and feeling at the same time. This is also true for embodied **listening.** Though it sounds so easy, it is actually challenging for most people to listen and feel their own bodily process within the same moment.

Exploring each of these practical aspects of contact can give us a path toward embodied relationship. These concrete functions provide the bodily ways that we can extend our own experience of embodiment into embodied relationship (see Box below).

PROXIMITY

The following exercise explores adjusting our proximity to others based on our bodily sensations.

> **Again, ground yourself in your own body. Be aware of the sensations and energy flow in your body. Have a friend stand about twenty feet away. Feel the sensations of response in your own body. Do you want to move toward your friend or further away? Allow yourself to do whichever you desire, following the sensational shifts in your body. Let yourself move into whatever proximity feels most satisfying in the moment. What happens if your friend shifts out of being still and moves according to his impulses?**

This is the dance of interaction that we mask by maintaining polite social distances. Often our sense of proximity to others can carry a great deal of

---

FIVE MODES OF EMBODIED CONTACT

Proximity

Touch

Eye Contact

Speaking

Listening

wounding, if as children we were not allowed to be as close to or as far away from others as we would like.

One young woman was surprised by what she found in this exercise. She was working with her relationship to her father, a relationship that she felt was suffocating. In exploring proximity, she discovered the process of setting a boundary was terrifying. She realized that she felt both suffocated *and* desperate for contact. When her partner got to a comfortable distance, she would rush forward, eyes wide in terror, put up her hands in a shielding gesture momentarily and then immediately grip her partner's hands.

Most of us are at least somewhat confused about comfortable proximity. Some situations may be more difficult than others. This varies from person to person. For some people, formal situations provide safe boundaries, whereas intimate situations are much more terrifying. For others the reverse is true. Experimenting with proximity in a laboratory-like situation can allow one to get comfortable with new possibilities. This can make real-life experiments easier. Finding a proximity that allows us to be in contact with ourselves and others at the same time is a powerful practice.

Experimenting with proximity can lead to awareness around positioning and facing in relation to other people. Do you want to be higher or lower, bigger or smaller, face to face, or side by side? Which relationships allow you to breathe more freely or circulate your energy more fully? The closest proximity we can have to another is to be touching.

EMBODIED TOUCH

Imagine the way babies respond when you touch them. Each touch engages the whole bodymind of the infant. The entire body moves in response to each touch. No touch is met with neutrality. Touching is a physical conversation.

Imagine conversely the way adults typically receive massage. We have been taught to be still to receive touch. Something in the adult shuts down to receive touch. We have taught that there is a clear delineation between giver and receiver.

When Margaret Mead, the anthropologist, visited the Samoan people in the 1950s, she was most struck by the amount of touching that occurred between them. She was convinced that the touching and bonding behaviors she saw in this so-called primitive people was a foundation for healthy individuals and relationships. She became a strong advocate for reconstructing our cultural attitudes toward touching.

In the late 1950s, Harry Harlow's psychological experiments with young monkeys and touch deprivation offered scientific evidence of the physical and psychological needs for touch in primates. While the implications of his research have continued to reverberate, our culture has moved slowly toward revamping our prohibitions against touch.

To practice embodied touch, respecting boundaries is paramount. To be able to say "yes," to touch, we first have to be able to say, "NO." Enduring a touch that you find uncomfortable is denying your body's natural intelligence.

 Practice with a friend having them touch you and telling them, "No, don't touch me," or "Don't touch me like that."

If we have been wounded or confused by touch, we may need to experience the possibility of being able to stop or redirect touch without being abandoned altogether.

Conversely, when we touch others, we may touch in a way that we think might please them. If pleasing the other is our entire strategy, touching becomes somewhat obligatory. The most sensually gratifying touch occurs when the person touching allows their body to touch out of their own internal impulses.

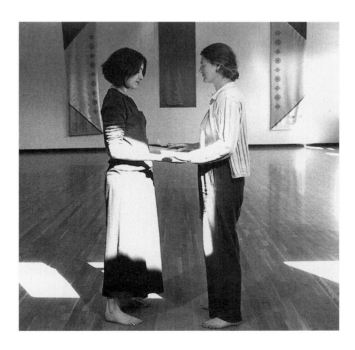

Embodying relationship with touch.

Feel this with yourself. Touch your face with your hands to relax your face. . . . Now, touch your face with your hands, however your hands want to touch. To do this, your hands wake up. They are more motivated, intelligent, and energized in their touching.

When toddlers or little children play together, they bring both of these touching exercises together. Imagine two young children touching each other. They explore the other out of raw curiosity. If one does something that the other doesn't like, they pull away, or say, "Don't," or push their friend's hand away. And then, they go right back to exploring.

Can you imagine two adults interacting so directly? Can you imagine yourself doing that? Embodied touch requires undoing many cultural lessons and truly redefining the nature of adult relationship. How can we embody the openness and healthy self-centeredness of toddlers and include the sensitivity and compassion of adulthood? Working with the endpoints is a good way to fine-tune one's relationship to both proximity and touch.

EYE CONTACT

The amount of communication that occurs via our eyes is so vast and subtle that it is beyond scientific measurement. In modern Western culture, we are very busy in our facial and hand gestures. This often serves as a smokescreen to hide our eyes. In visiting a pueblo in New Mexico, I saw, from a distance, two old women meet each other. They were walking toward each other and when they met, they stopped before each other. There was a syllable or two of greeting exchanged, and then their faces became still. Their arms hung by their sides. They stood looking into each other's eyes for a few moments. Then they leaned together briefly and continued on their ways. Watching them, I felt that I had witnessed something very simple and yet very extraordinary. I felt raw and thrilled.

Our eyes reveal so much of ourselves that it can be excruciating to really allow others to see us. Yet, in my psychotherapeutic work, I often find that seeing and being seen by others are among our most basic needs. The amount of time that newborn infants spend gazing into their mother's eyes is evidence of this need.

One of the most important pieces of advice that modern sexual counseling has to offer couples is the suggestion to work with eye contact while relating sexually. By making eye contact, we know that our partner is with us and we know a great deal about their internal experience.

 Spend some time moving and breathing in a way that brings you into contact with your own internal process. When you are ready, move across from a friend and practice continuing to move and

breathe while you are in eye contact. Let yourself move in and out of eye contact as you need to, but let the energy build. Generally, we avert our gazes out of embarrassment. Instead, feel the surge of energy that happens, and breathe and move as much as you need to stay in eye contact. Don't go for a fixed rigid gaze. This isn't a competition. But gently nudge yourself beyond your habitual comfort zone.

Working with relaxing our gaze, becoming willing to be seen and to see others more deeply is a powerful possibility. Recently I was speaking to a woman who facilitates interaction between dolphins and humans in the wild. I asked her what was the single most important aspect of these interactions. She said that when a dolphin looks at someone, they communicate deeply a healing feeling of love and connection. This is the potential of eye contact.

EMBODIED SPEECH

One of the most confusing experiences that children have with adults is when the words and the actions of the adult are not consonant. As adults we are challenged to say what we mean and mean what we say, or "to walk our talk." On the other hand, the adult skills of tact and diplomacy, often become

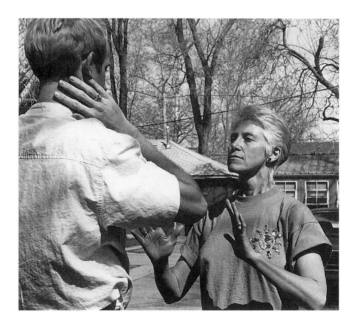

Embodying relationship with eye contact.

hastily given up for deceit. As we struggle to master these skills, it is easy for our attention to become stuck in an external focus.

We are often more concerned with social rules than with our internal energy flow. We conduct our interactions according to the rules of polite society. While we may find socially prescribed interactions sometimes less than satisfying, sometimes even confusing, we may not know how to change this. We may not know what would be more satisfying.

> *A young man was describing his experience of bringing his male lover to meet his family in a small town in Mississippi. The family had deep, but unspoken feelings against homosexual relationships. The interaction illustrates how confusing disembodied speech can be. His mother and aunts and their family friends were incredibly friendly to his lover in the way only upper class southern women can be: the more angry and disapproving they were, the nicer they acted. "Oh darlin', your career sounds so fascinatin' (read: disgusting). I can't imagine how excitin' it must be." And "You and my nephew must be so close to come all the way down here togetha . . . that's wonderful (read: I want to rip your throat out.)." The lover came away saying how well the visit had gone and wasn't it great they were so accepting. (How confusing "civilized" interactions can be.) Yet the mother and aunts might say, "I can't tell him how I really feel. That would be rude." Embodying our process in relationship can radically alter conventional social interactions.*

Embodied speech involves telling the truth, but it is more than that. Embodied speech refers to the ability to stay in touch with one's bodily experience while speaking, and to allow one's internal truth to sequence out through the body and into speech. This is a practice that requires much patience and ongoing development.

Embodied speaking often needs to begin with sounding as presented in the natural movement practice: letting go of your breath and voice so that simple utterances are not repressed. This most easily expands to basic words, "Yes," "No." From there simple sentences are often easiest to embody: "I like that," "I don't like that," "Come here," "Go away." Embodied speech stays in direct contact with the sensations that it is expressing, the words and the way they are spoken carrying the emotional tone and charge of those sensations. Generally most people need to slow way down and practice this with a great deal of attention. Initially, saying "Hi" in an embodied way might feel very intense.

Embodied speech can be very important in our relationship with ourselves. When a part of us feels denied and unexpressed, it ceases to participate. It can become stuck in its internal development. For example, if a part of us is still suffering from an early wound which the rest of us has worked to overcome, the wounded part may feel very unwelcome and abandoned. Truly healing this part would require letting it express itself and reintegrate into the rest of ourselves. An essential aspect of this is to let it speak for itself. The following exercise is intended to illustrate the process of embodying the speech of a particular internal aspect of oneself.

> **Try this exercise with two other people. Imagine they speak different languages and you are acting as an interpreter between them. Let one of the people tell you in private something they would like to say to the other person. Now leave that person and walk over to the other person to communicate the message.**
>
> **Now try it again. This time hold your partner's hand and walk together to the other person. Look and listen to your partner in the presence of the third person. As you repeat what your partner said, try to match some of his gestures and intonations. As you speak, look back and forth between the two people.**

How do these two experiences feel different? Often when we talk we convey our inner experience in the manner of the first trial, with lots of distance between our bodily experience and our words. How does the quality and effectiveness of our communication change when we practice sequencing from our inner experience to our speech? Imagine communicating within a situa-

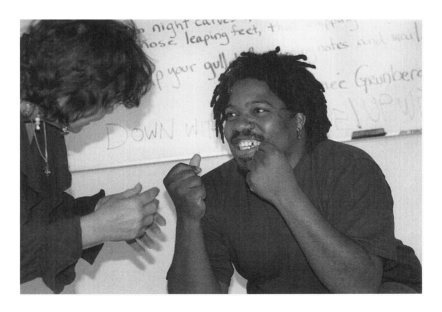

Embodying relationship while speaking.

tion of apparent conflict. In a distanced communication one might just say: "I don't agree." If we attempt to embody our process and speak from there, the same communication might go more in this direction. "Whew. I feel tense . . . (big exhale) . . . I know this isn't working for me. I would really prefer to try it this way."

In communicating with others about our emotions, speaking from a body-based position can facilitate clarity. Consider the difference between saying, "I feel a great longing for such and such," and " I think it would be good if such and such happened." Embodied speaking can also deepen a communication. For example, consider the statement, "I'm frightened of this. The idea of it makes me quivery in my legs," versus "I don't think it's a good idea."

In a training seminar for professional health care workers, the participants were practicing embodied listening and speaking in dyads. One member of the group was feeling quite emotional and this person's partner responded in a simple way that felt so honest and embodied that it has stayed with me ever since. He said, "You know . . . I don't really know you at all, but at this moment, I feel I really care about you." These words could have been said in a very empty, stylized way; however, this person was thoroughly resting on his feet. His eyes were remarkably open and soft. His posture was so unaffected that his words felt thoroughly believable. These simple words communicated profoundly.

Learning to embody speech is an ongoing process that seems to be able to deepen continually. Practice on your own first and then with someone whom you feel to be nonthreatening. This can lay the ground for embodied speech even in uncomfortable situations.

 Spend a few moments in natural movement until you feel fairly awake and alive in your body. Pick a particular aspect of your life that you are sorting through and have a lot of feelings about. First allow yourself to make sounds as you attend to your feelings and thoughts about this issue. Keep breathing and moving. Next, speak simple phrases of what you are thinking. Keep breathing and moving and continuing to sound. Work your way up to speaking a full sentence and then to being able to describe the whole issue. Always the questions to ask along the way are "Am I still feeling my body? Is my energy still sequencing?" If not, come back to natural movement.

EMBODIED LISTENING

Embodied speech is much easier for most people than embodied listening. Yet both involve the same process. The task is how to listen to someone else and feel my own internal bodily process at the same time. The trick is that if we are really listening, we are touched by what we hear. This changes our internal process.

Often in the helping professions, people are concerned about taking on too much from other people's lives. Obviously, it is important to learn not to become over-involved. One of the best ways to do this is to "stay in your own body." Keep feeling your own body and allowing its internal energy to circulate.

On the other hand, when we are deeply feeling our bodies, our perceptual processes deepen. Imagine the difference between closing your eyes and listening to a symphony versus rushing past an orchestra on your way to somewhere else. In the first scenario, the music enters your system more deeply. I tell my psychotherapy students that once something is in their bodies, to consider it their own.

So, embodied listening can be a way to differentiate from others, in that you can recognize your own internal experience. It can also be a way to become more empathetic, to listen more deeply with more of yourself. Doing this can require strengthening your concepts of who you are and how you are separate from whomever you are listening to.

To practice embodied listening spend some time moving and breathing, feeling your body. When you feel firmly rooted in your own physical experience, ask someone to speak with you about something that is very important to them. The more moving the story is the better it will be for the exercise. Ask their permission that you continue to move and breathe as you listen. As you listen, keep coming back to your own bodily experience. Keep giving your internal process permission to flow within you. Notice how the communication of the other person affects you internally.

We have been taught that fixed attention is the only kind of attention. In school, we are taught to sit still with our eyes fixed upon our teacher. Often that is not really a good way to absorb new information. This is especially true for most children under the age of seven, for whom it is neurologically impossible to think without moving and vocalizing.

I had a student who would, from time to time, become seemingly transfixed by what I was saying. He would stare at me in a way that looked fascinated to an extreme. It was a bit disconcerting. Finally, I asked him what was going on during these times. As he explored the experience, he realized that he was totally distracted at those moments and not hearing a thing. As a young student in Catholic school, he had learned to avoid punishment for not paying attention by seeming really attentive when he was actually daydreaming. I think this is true for many of us. Much of what masquerades as attentive listening is actually a facade.

I have found many benefits of allowing myself to stay with my own internal process while listening. I have much more energy and curiosity about what others are saying. I find more meaning in what I am hearing. I notice more quickly when there is a discrepancy between the words and the actions of the person speaking.

All of the practices of embodied relationship point in the same direction: how to be with oneself fully and truly in contact with another at the same time. To inspire this journey, imagine a young child stepping expectantly into a new environment, eager to explore: eyes are open and shining, looking all around; mouth is relaxed and slightly open; hands are extended a bit. All of these gestures add up to a position of being available to engage. How often do you see adults initiate relationship from this open stance?

The basic skill here is to stay in your body while interacting with the world. The possibility is to trust and allow your own naturally intelligent responses to the world around you. Simple body-based approaches can facilitate this: using your endpoints to monitor touch and proximity, and taking the time to embody your process as you speak and listen. Generally, these practices require very sensitive and repeated trials to unlearn habits of distancing from ourselves and others. This is because our cultural biases affect us so strongly and unconsciously. In order to embody relationship, it is important to become conscious of our cultural conditioning.

Spirit and the Body

Our bodies not only bespeak our emotions, but also allow us to connect with spirit. Perhaps the most profound relationship in our lives is our relationship with the spiritual world. This can be deeply satisfying when it is embodied. Our bodily responses alert us to what is wonderful and miraculous. It is the body that sends the message "Go toward that." Having diminished our experience of aliveness, we seem to no longer remember that a naturally intelligent body is also spiritually inhabited. Entrenched in polarities, body and spirit are regarded as conflicting realms, and paying attention to the body in a way that would honor its inherent messages is too often considered to be a materialistic distraction from the spiritual realm. A seminal belief in the field of somatic psychology is that by enlivening our bodies we *feel* spirit. We are in contact with the deepest aspect of the world. Through embodying our natural intelligence, we allow spirit to incarnate ever more fully, and we feel this visitation at a cellular level.

I imagine Moses in the desert, praying for his prophesies. I breathe. Feeling the image in my body, my heart rises. The surge continues upward, welling up into my throat with a longing that expresses itself out through my mouth and eyes. They reach upward. Even my hands open up and out.

As I imagine the Buddha sitting under the bodhi tree, achieving enlightenment, my eyes soften and rest back in their sockets. The top of my head awakens. A deep breath releases my diaphragm. A feeling of openness slides down the front of my sacrum.

On the most simple level, when we have connected to a source of spiritual renewal, such as prayer, meditation, ritual, or experience in nature, our bodies will crave that. We will feel refreshed and energized. Likewise, our bodies also tell us when spirit is not being tapped. I once attended a wedding in an exquisitely beautiful Catholic church. Its hand-painted ceiling invited us up and up and up. The golden tapestries sparkled. The coolness of the wooden pews suggested silence and simplicity. Entering this space, I felt a moment of possibility. As the priest began his amplified discourse about movies, magazines, and marriage, the promise of the space dissipated. I felt compressed and numb. I felt out of contact.

In this instance the human activity was not resonating with the fullness of the potential spirit. Relationship with spirit was not happening. Moments like this can lead us to the conclusion that certain religions or spiritual practices are empty.

Organized religions tend to regard the body as a temptation to be rebuked, a distraction to be ignored, or a burden to be transcended. It seems clear, though, that when we are not alive in our bodies, spiritual values like union, compassion, and sacred view become concepts without a living, breathing manifestation. *I remember the first time, at two years old, that I consciously noticed the stars. As that memory visits me now my heart rises forward and up with a feeling of mists parting in front of it. A very rich, broad breath comes with it. My nostrils flare, my pelvic floor pulsates. This was my first moment of being conscious of the heavens.*

In the same way that abstracting emotions induces us to *not* feel, conceptualizing spirituality robs us of the possibility for transcendent experience.

Embodied spirituality may be seen as a connection between feelings of aliveness in the body and some mental attitude that connects that aliveness to a larger sense of the world. An example of this would be experiencing a deep, cleansing breath at the end of a prayer. If the one who prays believes that the breath connects with the cosmos, then a cycle is created. A concept of spirituality that includes a sensate dimension increases aliveness. Aliveness can expand the concept.

Definite bodily shifts occur when we acknowledge a larger perspective. Important spiritual perspectives that resonate with a somatic approach might include an understanding of each person's basic goodness and wholeness, a sense of the vastness of pain in the world, recognition of the sacredness of all of life and nature, and acknowledgment that on an ultimate level there is fundamentally no wound or problem to be fixed. It is interesting to compare bodily experiences as you reflect on a given situation from various stances, ones that move progressively from a more narrow, personal view to a wider perspective of spiritual connection.

Imagine a situation in which you perceive some pain or difficulty in the life of someone close to you. Take a moment to breathe, opening your awareness to the situation. Now worry about it. Feel your mental distress about the situation permeate your consciousness. What happens in you body as you adopt a worrying stance?

Now bring awareness to your breath again, and let go of worrying. How does your body shift?

Take another moment to breathe. Now engage an attitude of concern. Feel your own mix of interest in and apprehension for the well-being of your friend. What happens in your body as you adopt a concerned stance? How are your sensations of concern different from those of worry? In what ways are they the same?

Bringing awareness to your breath, let go of your concern. Explore sympathy, empathy, and compassion each in a similar way, paying attention to the bodily sensations accompanying each state of consciousness.

In my experience, compassion is the state of consciousness that provides me with the largest perspective. Compassion allows me to be in the fullest contact with myself and other. Sitting with a person in pain, I experience empathy. My heart moves forward, two invisible hands gently pressing it toward the other person. My eyes focus, pupils constrict slightly, brow gently furrows. This creates a particular stance.

Opening my awareness to include the inherently correct nature of all situations, I become aware of the person's basic health, recognizing the pain they are in is temporary and in no way damages that basic wellness. This view opens me up to compassion rather than empathy. I breathe. The slight pressure around my heart releases. My breath moves up into my shoulders. My eyes move apart. Weight falls fully into my belly. I shift into a more compassionate stance.

Cognitive attitudes affect our physical experiences. When the body's process is connected with spiritual intentions, feelings of aliveness move out of the body and into contact with the world. Conversely, perceptions of the world penetrate into the core of the body when one has an embodied experience of spirituality.

Stanley Keleman, author of *Emotional Anatomy* and a leader in the field of somatic psychology, gave a talk entitled "The Body as Meditation" at the

1992 Body Psychology Symposium at the Naropa Institute in Boulder, Colorado. This passage from Keleman's talk illustrates his experience of the connection between the individual body and a larger sense of spirit.

> *I took a boat ride on the lake of Lucerne in Switzerland. Everybody knows the Swiss have a big navy—these little steamboats electrically driven, mostly, that go up and down on the lake. You get on these boats and shake, rattle, and roll, and they are not very good at dealing with the minor waves they create, let alone the wind swells.*
>
> *I get on the boat and I realize that the beat of the engine has got a particular rhythm. That this engine is moving in its own mechanical way—putt putt putt boom putt putt putt—and there's a rhythmicity to it, and that I enjoy just standing and letting the rhythm of this boat move through me.*
>
> *Then I realize that there's a rhythm that has nothing to do with this. This realization adds a second level—being in the water. This boat is going up and down, right? And it's also shaking in its own way. Then I have these two patterns of riding up and down and being jiggled back and forth. Then I realize, "Hey, wait a second. I myself am going in and out—boom boom. What is this?" And so I pay attention to going in and out. Then I notice, "Hey, wait a second. I am not standing here on this ship, just as some package with a tight boundary. I mean, I'm moving into my environment and I'm moving back."*
>
> *The sea of Lucerne is surrounded by the Swiss Alps, so it's like a big body, like a big container, like a big outer boundary. And I am pulsing in an environment that is pulsating, even though it has boundaries—the mountains. I am now in a big pulsating environment. I watch this big flock of birds take off and as they begin to move through this air, gliding, I realize they're pulsating. It is not a straight glide, but it's a pulsatory movement within a pulsatory movement. I turn to look at my friends and I see that we are moving, moving in and out and changing shape. I see them in a way that I have never experienced them before, different qualities of them. One could say that I see their real shapes rather than their social shapes.*
>
> *I then recognize and I experience that I'm in an eternal sea of continual pulsing patterns, and this is a bodying pattern. From the beginning of my existence I am in something and it's pulsing me, bodying me. And it is bodied.*

In Keleman's view enlightenment is a state of feeling the pulsations of the world fully. Our internal pulsations and the pulsations around us create a constant dialogue that can amplify our sensitivity to energy. By feeling the rhythms and cycles of the world, we feel ourselves more clearly. By feeling ourselves more fully, we receive more from the world. In this way we learn both about our bonds with the world and our individuality. The issue of union with the world and individuality is an essential spiritual paradox that comes together within the body. Dealt with conceptually, this paradox is tricky to resolve. The bodily experience, however, is simple and concrete.

When my individual experience comes together with a sense of the vastness of the world, both its pain and its sacredness, I feel very erect. My heart and face soften with a minute sob as I exhale. My skin tingles. I feel deep into my womb and heart.

When I take this state out into the world, I am deeply touched by the people, animals, and plants I move past. My perceptions of them are received into the depths of my trunk; my muscles quietly ripple in recognition. My inner responses move freely out to the periphery of my body, becoming silently, energetically communicative.

One could speculate that human beings instinctively seek energetically communicative states. All animals, including humans, motivate toward full bodily aliveness and express that in relationship. Our human potential gives us the opportunity to both embody the unity of aliveness that is shared by all beings *and* to be aware of that unity as both concept and experience. This somatic definition of spiritual process does not polarize the animal nature and the higher self. Rather, both are considered essential elements to full spiritual embodiment. Let us celebrate the fullest possible relationship between body and spirit.

Personal Inquiry and Explorations

Flowing from the inside out:

How do you share what is inside you with others? How much of you do you feel you are able to share with others? Do you feel satisfied by this? Do you feel resigned about it? What are particular kinds of situations which seem pertinent, either positively or negatively, to your ability to express your internal experience? Do you tend to get stuck in internally focused states and have difficulty communicating?

Flowing from the outside in:

How do you get what you need or want from the world around you? Are you able to take in what is available to you? Do you feel satisfied by this? Do you feel resigned about it? What are particular kinds of situations which seem pertinent, either positively or negatively, to your ability to receive from the outside world? Do you tend to get stuck in externally focused states and have difficulty coming back to your own experience?

Sit by yourself for periods of time. Feel the flow of your breath in and out through your body. Relax your posture. Gently let your attention shift from aspects of your internal experience to aspects of the world around you. Imagine a flowing connection between yourself and the outside world. When you feel somewhat comfortable with this, practice it in a variety of situations:

- in nature
- in some environment which is important to you spiritually, such as a church, a temple, a shrine, or a special place.
- with a person you love.
- with a person with whom you feel in conflict.

CHAPTER 4

Energetic Development: Pathways of Life and Pathways of Movement

Development does not occur in a linear progression but as overlapping waves with each pattern being integrated and modified by the emergence of new patterns. Eventually all patterns are contained in each of the others as an expressive element or as a shadow support.

—Bonnie Bainbridge

THE ENERGY OF LIFE IS FLOWING THROUGH US ALL THE TIME. THIS PROCESS BOTH MOVES AND SHAPES ALL ORGANISMS. WHEN INTERACTING WITH ADULTS, IT IS EASY TO SEE HOW THEY HAVE BEEN SHAPED BY THEIR LIVES. THIS CHAPTER EXAMINES THE SPECIFIC WAYS IN WHICH ENERGY SHAPES OUR DEVELOPMENT. TO HELP US UNDERSTAND THE PATHWAYS ALONG WHICH WE ARE SHAPED, WE CAN OBSERVE THE CIRCULATION OF ENERGY THROUGH THE ENDPOINTS OF THE BODY AS DISCUSSED IN CHAPTER 2, THESE ARE THE HANDS, FEET, HEAD, AND PERINEUM (IDENTIFIED HERE AS THE PELVIC FLOOR). THE MAIN PORTALS THROUGH WHICH ENERGY COMES AND GOES IN THE BODY, THE ENDPOINTS DEMARCATE THE MAJOR PATHWAYS OF MOVEMENT SEQUENCES THROUGH THE BODY.

✻　✻　✻

While traffic flow along these pathways varies from moment to moment, each individual has basic patterns and preferences that persist over time. Some people's hands are naturally more active in circulating energy, while other people may be more feet-oriented. These differences can be either innate and learned. One can observe major differences in energy flow even between newborns. Beyond our innate patterns, we are strongly influenced by our mother's energy flow in utero, and later by that of our family and our culture. Particular experiences, such as our birth experience, physical accidents, or emotional trauma, may greatly affect these patterns as well.

Underlying our individual patterns of energy flow, both learned and innate, are universal patterns. There are many systems which study energy flow through the body. The meridian systems of oriental medicine and the systems underlying various types of bodywork that focus on our energy fields, such as polarity therapy, are two major examples. All these systems are related because the body has a basic truth. The approach taken here is based primarily on studies of early motor development and the study of the evolutionary origins of movement. While these motor patterns have been studied by many different physical therapists and biologists, much of the specific approach here is based on Body-Mind Centering, the work of Bonnie Bainbridge Cohen. To that I have added a more in-depth look at the psychological aspects of these movements.

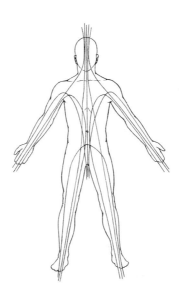

Pathways connecting each of the endpoints.

Studies of early motor development in humans reveal a universal set of movements through which infants generally, though individualistically, proceed during the first year or so of life. These actions, which can be considered building blocks for all movement, have an internal neurological integrity manifesting as a hierarchy of stages.

This hierarchy can be observed in animals as well. Evolutionarily, fish evolved before amphibians, which preceded reptiles, which preceded mammals. Fish use *spinal movement* to locomote. Amphibians move with their upper limbs as one unit and their lower limbs as an opposing unit. Imagine a frog jumping: the differentiation is between the upper and lower halves of the body. This amphibious type of movement is called *homologous movement*. Reptilian movement differentiates the two sides of the body. Imagine a lizard climbing a rock: each side moves in unison with itself, and in opposition to the other side. This is called *homolateral movement*. Mammalian movement sequences diagonally across the body, one arm paired with the opposite leg. This is called *contralateral movement*.

The human child reiterates these evolutionary stages. Initially, the newborn uses primarily spinal movements. Most infants soon adds homologous movements to push up. Soon after some homolateral movements are explored. These eventually lead to various kinds of locomoting with the belly on the ground. Out of this contralateral crawling develops, which eventually leads to standing and walking. An infant's early motor development consists of these basic neurological actions derived from our evolutionary heritage. Each of these actions will be discussed thoroughly in the pages that follow. They consist of either pushing or reaching with all of the endpoints of the body. Since the endpoints are characterized by the highest concentration of sensory nerve endings and the finest motoric capacity, they are the parts of the body most easily equipped to communicate with the outside world, both in terms of receptivity and responsivity. To illustrate this, try a simple experiment.

 Look around your environment and pick a somewhat intricately shaped object. Trace the shape of this object with your index finger. Now trace the same shape with your elbow.

This should clearly show the endpoints' greater capacity for precision. Another important aspect of the endpoints is that their movement has an integrated coordination within the body. Try this experiment.

 Let your arms rest down along your sides. Sense the tips of your fingers. Feeling the tips of your fingers, allow them to reach up into the space above. As they continue above your head, feel what musculature is involved in the movement. Now return your arms to your sides.

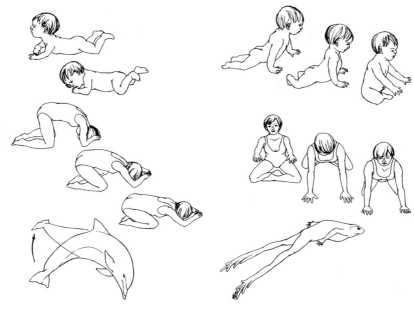

Spinal movement.   Homologous movement.

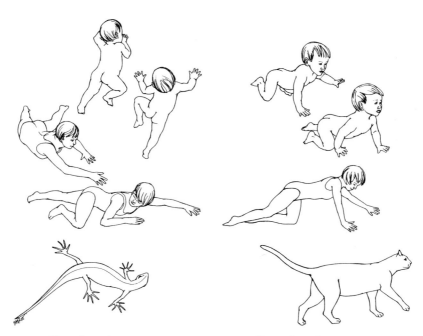

Homolateral movement.   Contralateral movement.

This time feel your elbow, and let it lead the movement. Again, feel what musculature is involved.

This should illustrate that when the endpoints (in this case, the fingertips) lead the movement, the muscular sequence is complete and continuous. Integrated movement is movement in which the moving and supporting body are working as a whole. This occurs when the initiation of the movement is from an endpoint. When the elbow leads, the forearm remains passively uninvolved. It is not integrated into this movement.

Overall, movement initiated at the endpoints is more sensitive to the environment and fully coordinated within the body. If we feel in ourselves or observe in others that a gesture with the arms is not fully articulated in the hands, then we might presume that it has not yet been fully processed; that is, that the inner process is not yet fully in contact with the environment. Imagine someone gesticulating angrily with relatively limp hands. The internal process of anger is not fully in contact with the environment. In almost all important human processes, the relationship between the inner and the outer world is key. Working with movement sequencing in and out through the endpoints of the body is a graphic way to address this relationship. We can characterize movement that sequences to or from the endpoints as more alert, sensitive, vulnerable, and capable, both in perceiving and acting.

We are constantly giving and receiving through our endpoints—giving and receiving objects, information, love, energy, anger, and so forth. Neurologically this flow of giving and receiving occurs through five fundamental actions of either *yielding, pushing, reaching, grasping, or pulling.* Play for a moment with your hand in space and in contact with various objects around you. Whatever your hand does is some variation or combination of these five actions.

Five Fundamental Actions

YIELDING

Yielding, the least obvious of the five fundamental actions, underlies the others. Yielding is a quality of resting in contact. It is not resting inertly, which is resting out of contact.

Rest your hand on an object and feel it. In feeling it, there may be a sense of flow, of being in contact. Withdraw this sense. Now reengage it. You are playing with your ability to yield. For a more pronounced sense of yielding, stand up and contract all your muscles, then release them and feel a sense of yielding into gravity.

There are different ways of yielding. One can yield into a physical force,

```
╔══════════════════════════════════════════╗
║                                            ║
║         FIVE FUNDAMENTAL ACTIONS           ║
║                                            ║
║                Yielding                    ║
║                                            ║
║                Pushing                     ║
║                                            ║
║                Reaching                    ║
║                                            ║
║                Grasping                    ║
║                                            ║
║                Pulling                     ║
║                                            ║
╚══════════════════════════════════════════╝
```

such as gravity, as above, or the force of being pushed by another body. One can yield to internal impulses rather than inhibiting them. Imagine the feeling of your eyes welling up with tears, allowing yourself to cry.

One can also allow an internal part of the body to yield into its natural shape, rhythm, or position. Entertain the possibility that some of your internal organs are either cramped or sagging. Breathe into your trunk and find an area that has some discomfort that might relate to this. Visualize that area yielding into itself. Like a sea sponge plumping up with fluid, it assumes its rightful shape and position, even vibration. This is the most subtle form of yielding.

Yielding brings us into contact with the environment so that we can feel if we want to push or reach or pull. When your hand is resting on an object without a sense of contact, it is not yielding—your hand is instead out of contact with the environment. To a greater or lesser degree, there is no energy sequencing through your hand.

Yielding underlies our basic relationship to the world. In utero and as young infants, we do a great deal of yielding. These early experiences with yielding affect our relationship to yielding throughout our lives. Yielding has to do with what we might describe as "letting down," or feeling safe. Yielding is about just *being in contact*, not doing. We all have some confusion about yielding. I have never met someone who was able to fully yield in all the endpoints and along all their pathways.

Our ability to yield is the basis for our ability to take effective action in the world. If we are not in contact with our environment, we are not able to assess it accurately. In yielding there is a release of weight into our environment; we physically rest our weight into that which we are in contact with. This weight serves as a springboard from which to push away, just as a diver yields down into the diving board before pushing off it and then reaching into

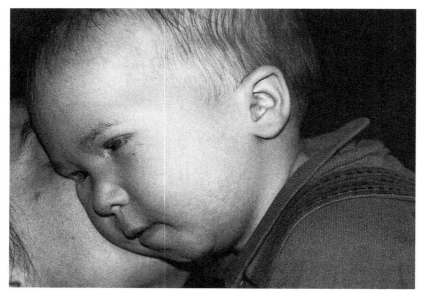

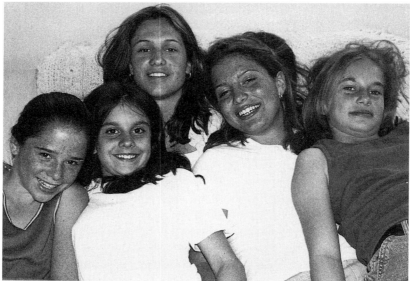

Yielding into contact.

space. In this way yielding is the basis for pushing, and then reaching, grasping or pulling.

Healing our relationship to yielding involves observing when we are doing it and when we are not. Observing where in our bodies we are yielding furthers this. As I write this I am frequently conscious of my throat, which gets over-involved in this writing. I am trying to speak what I am thinking. Inviting my throat to yield brings greater ease to the flow between my brain and hands, the two aspects of my body that are the primary actors in the writing process.

Often, healing our relationship to yielding brings up a great deal of fear. It feels unsafe to let down. I have found that the earth is very safe for most people to yield into. It is so solid and reliable, so much bigger than us, always there, unconditional. Lying with one's belly on the earth can be a way of healing the earliest experiences of yielding, as once again, our umbilicus is connected to the mother.

PUSHING

As we saw with the diver, yielding underlies pushing. Pushing is the most basic of our actions. Unlike yielding, pushing is an act of separating ourselves from the immediate environment. The environment is our springboard for moving out into new spaces.

A push is an action that concentrically contracts (shortens) all the musculature around the pushing limb. This contraction occurs in degrees, the push compressing the body inward from the endpoint. This compression or condensation integrates the body around the pushing (weight-bearing) surface. By integration, I mean that it organizes the movement into a coordinated unit focused on one action. When the body is organized around a push, that push can either support or move the body. You can experience this directly by doing the following exploration:

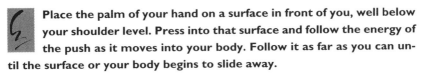
Place the palm of your hand on a surface in front of you, well below your shoulder level. Press into that surface and follow the energy of the push as it moves into your body. Follow it as far as you can until the surface or your body begins to slide away.

As we push, we literally become denser, more substantial. Pushing illuminates the fullness of the body. Psychologically this means feeling ourselves, our boundaries, our ability to maintain boundaries, and our ability to support ourselves. The power of the push allows us to feel empowered. We can differentiate between what's "in here" and what's "out there." As the infant pushes with both hands, she separates from mother or from the supporting surface.

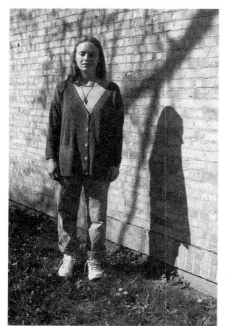

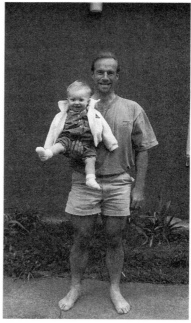

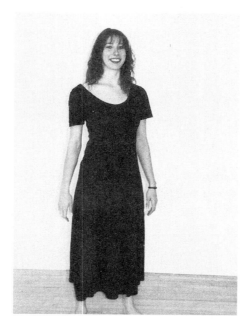

Even in simply standing, the various qualities of yield,
push, and reach can be expressed.

This develops into a way of saying "no." We push away from what we don't want.

As adults, the extent to which we are able to push reflects our internal sense of support, individuation, confidence, and ability to propel ourselves. Pushing gives us a sense of "being able to stand on our own two feet," "sticking up for ourselves," not being "a pushover."

REACHING

Reach, on the other hand, is an action that lengthens the musculature around the reaching limb. As our endpoints become alert to something "out there" and move toward it, there is a sense of release through the reaching part.

 Place your hand on the same surface as before. Become aware of its texture beneath your skin. Let your hand reach forward as it explores the texture. Feel the sense of lightness in the hand and arm as the energy of the reach moves inward from the hand.

There is literally a lessening of proprioceptive input as we reach out. Proprioceptors are the nerve endings that give us information about ourselves. As we reach, our attention is focused externally. Reaching is the way we extend out into space, toward others, toward objects. It is our ability to go beyond ourselves. Psychologically, reaching manifests curiosity, desire, longing, compassion. Imagine the moment in which a brightly colored object catches an infant's eye. The hand begins to move slowly, with complete attention toward the object. The infant has no sense of when the connection will happen, so the reach is continuous and full of life and curiosity.

To support a reach out into the environment, there must be adequate push to maintain the original position. To illustrate this, imagine an infant in a newly gained hands-and-knees position. The infant is drawn to an object in front and reaches a hand out toward it, but because there is not adequate push through the other arm, the infant collapses to the floor. With time, the push becomes stronger and can support the reach. Push precedes reach. Support precedes movement.

Just as the infant reaches into the unknown, as adults, reaching takes us out of the known and into the new. As adults our ability to reach allows us to invite others, reach out with compassion, envision a goal. This might be accompanied by a sense of vulnerability, groundlessness, or riskiness. For adults as well as infants, the ability to reach depends on the support of the push. Without push, reach becomes a falling toward, a tumble into chaos; a reach to another may become a demand for external support. Without the supporting push, there is no ground from which to move out. Often an inability to reach is rooted in an inability to push, or a prohibition against pushing. Here the developmental hierarchy gives guidance as to the path for further development. When a reach is supported, it can be the exciting connection of inner and outer worlds.

GRASPING AND PULLING

Yielding precedes pushing, and pushing precedes reaching. Likewise reaching can blossom into grasping and pulling. As we reach out into space and come in contact with something outside of us, if we are pleased with it we often

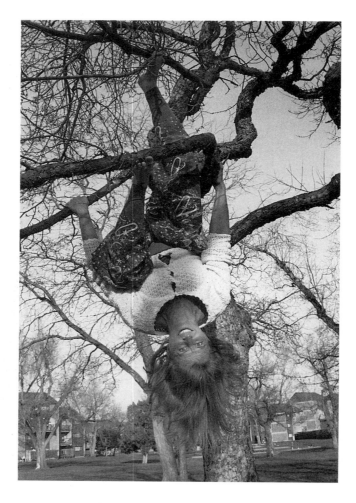

Grasping with the feet and hands.

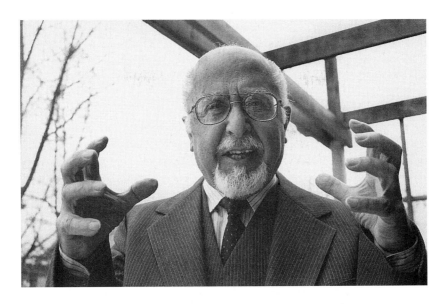

Even without an object, the quality of grasping
is expressed in this man's face and hands.

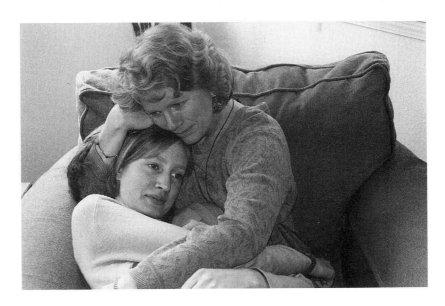

After reaching, grasping, and pulling,
one can return to a state of yield in order to receive.

would like to bring it closer to ourselves, or bring us closer to it. We do this by grasping and pulling. Again, imagine an infant reaching for something bright and moving. Contact is made. Quickly, she grasps it and pulls it toward her mouth. Imagine a monkey reaching toward a vine. He reaches it, grasps it, and pulls his body through space toward it.

Psychologically, our ability to grasp and pull relies on our abilities to yield, push, and reach. If we are not able to reach toward what we want, we may never have the opportunity to grasp it and take it into ourselves. On the other hand, overusing our ability to grasp and pull limits our ability to receive in a satisfying way. In an unsatisfying pattern, we do not sequence from the grasping/pulling endpoint into our core. Thus, there is no satisfaction, and we feel the need to grasp and pull again.

Conversely, it is possible to reverse the direction. Out of fear or anger, we can pull away from the world into ourselves. This action becomes tangled up within us and makes sequencing other actions difficult. Again, satisfying giving and receiving becomes blocked.

 Look around your environment for something you want. Feel your body and breathe. Allow yourself to reach toward the thing you are wanting, grasp it, and pull it toward you. Bring it to the midline of your body. If it is something to smell, bring it to your nose. If it is something to taste, bring it to your mouth. If it is something to receive emotionally, bring it to your throat or heart or belly. Allow yourself to feel the experience of receiving it.

Neurological Organization

As mentioned previously, the neurological organization of movement precedes from spinal to homologous to homolateral to contralateral. We see this both evolutionarily (fish to amphibians to reptiles to mammals) and in human motor development. The human infant in utero is a completely and choicelessly integrated unit; there is no neurological differentiation. A stimulus to any part of the body elicits a total body response. We can all picture the digestive squirming of a newborn—even her face seems to be digesting. The whole body digests in unison.

Slowly, with time, body parts begin to differentiate out of this pattern. They begin to be able to perform actions that do not involve the whole body. Initially, the head begins to make movements independent of the rest of the body. This develops into spinal movement. Then both hands begin to make movements independent of the feet, and vice versa. This is homologous movement, like the frog. Here the hands are still responding together to the same stimulus. As one hand (or one foot) differentiates and begins to move independent of the other, we reach the homolateral level of neurological organization, like the lizard. At this level, movement sequences up or down one side of the body. Finally, mammalian movement (contralateral) begins with one hand (or foot) and proceeds diagonally across the body to the opposite foot (or hand).

The progression through these levels is not linear, though each previous level supports and facilitates the next. In other words, you don't "graduate" from one neurological level, leaving behind the more primitive ones. Without an ongoing spinal connection, no amount of pushing in the lizards' limbs would lift his head from dragging on the ground. At the level of contralateral movement, all the previous levels are active and supporting.

These basic neurological actions form the building blocks for adult human movement. Picture an infant nuzzling his mother's breast in search of the nipple. The action is composed of a series of small pushes and reaches initiated from the nose, mouth, and cheek. In this way we learn to move our heads and subsequently our spines. This small action becomes enlarged until it has the power to draw the whole body into movement. Picture an older infant on hands and knees. A sound issues from behind the infant, who reaches first from the ear, then from the eyes, and then from the entire head in an action that moves the spine and then completes itself in a series of steps that turn the whole body. The reach from the head is part of this movement of crawling to turn around. Like all the basic actions, it is one of the building blocks that forms adult movement. An adult who is drawn to a sound would use this action as part of walking toward it.

Twelve Basic Neurological Actions

The following discussion of the major developmental actions is designed to introduce the reader to the actions and some of their psychological manifestations. They will be presented in an order that somewhat reflects our movement development. However, the reader must realize that in the actual development of any individual, many tracks are being cultivated at once; therefore, any single linear track cannot fully represent the course of development.

SPINAL PUSH FROM THE HEAD

The spinal push from the head is the basic neurological action that we use to do a headstand, to push out of the birth canal, to burrow under a pillow, or simply to support the weight of our head on our body. These are just a few examples. To experience a spinal push from the head, try the following:

Sitting or standing in a vertical position, place both hands on your head. Allow your body to slump down under the weight of your hands. Now, feeling the surface of your head under your hands, push with your head into your hands. Continue until your body feels full and upright again, as opposed to squashed and slumped as it did before. Repeat this as needed to clarify the action and the feelings.

Pushing from the head allows us to sequence energy from the trunk out through the head. The spine being the core of the body, any emotional reactions that occur in the trunk (that is, in the viscera or the endocrine system) must be processed within the pathway of spinal movement. Psychologically, we might say that pushing from the head establishes the internal space for core processes. This action is a basic assertion of one's right to occupy space with one's inner experience.

In *The Evolutionary Origins of Movement* (1986), Bonnie Bainbridge Cohen describes this action as "stimulating proprioceptive knowledge of one's self, developing the base for the establishment of one's personal kinosphere, and developing one's mind of inner attention." Subjectively we might experience this pattern as one associated with self-containment, and with being as opposed to doing.

TWELVE BASIC NEUROLOGICAL ACTIONS

Spinal Push from the Head

Spinal Push from the Pelvic Floor

Homologous Push from the Hands

Homologous Push from the Feet

Homolateral Push from the Hand

Homolateral Push from the Foot

Spinal Reach from the Head

Spinal Reach from the Pelvic Floor

Homologous Reach from the Hands

Homologous Reach from the Feet

Contralateral Reach from the Hand

Contralateral Reach from the Foot

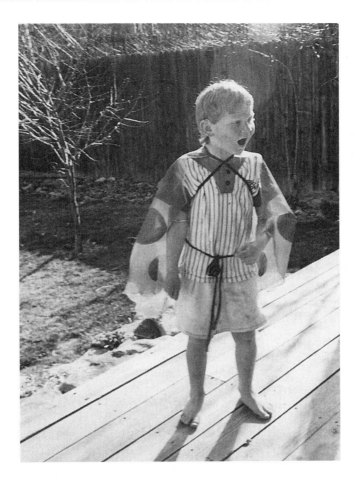

Spinal push from the head.

To illustrate how this action might arise developmentally, let's consider Jane, a young woman who complained of feeling "stuck" in a live-in relationship. She was struggling with wanting to move out and not wanting to hurt her partner. She experienced great difficulty in finishing sentences relating to moving out. When Jane spoke of this possibility she would contort her face, constrict her throat, clench her jaw, vigorously push on her forehead, and lightly bang the back of her head on the wall behind her. Clearly she was illustrating an inability to sequence a push out through her head, which paralleled her inability to tell her partner that she would like to move out. She experienced the physical pattern as feeling "held back" or "squashed" with her head, neck, and upper chest.

In her frustration, Jane burrowed her head into a pillow. I encouraged her to feel *herself pushing into it. Pushing from the head is essential in the process of being born; recalling the pattern often evokes birth issues. This definitely seemed to be the case here, as that bit of pressure into the pillow (which might have re-evoked the pressure of the cervix, birth canal, or perineum) immediately intensified her breathing which led to crying and some choking. Initially, the feeling was one of helplessness to meet the pressure and grief about that helplessness. As I pressed into the pillow responsively to her breath, shifting the area I was pressing against and the degree of pressure, she was gradually able to connect to her ability to push through. This process continued for approximately ten minutes, accompanied by crying, moaning, and grunting. Eventually Jane pushed "through," her push sequencing all the way through her head rather than imploding in the neck, facial muscles, or soft tissues of the head. She experienced a sense of release and said that she felt different. In subsequent sessions, she connected this new and different feeling with allowing her needs to be honored. As a result of this process, Jane was able to verbally express to her partner her need to move out, which she eventually did.*

In this case, the spinal push from the head was associated with the protection of basic personal needs. As it often does, the action seemed associated with a birth experience. Other clients have experienced this action in relation to issues such as "a right to be here" or "confidence in the ability to survive." However, it is not possible to formulaically categorize certain issues with each of the basic neurological actions. Rather, as in this case, it is necessary to see how the body expresses an emotional struggle and then respond to that in the present.

SPINAL PUSH FROM THE PELVIC FLOOR

This action is a bit more tricky to approach, as the pelvic floor—or perineum—is ignored in this culture. Yet, from a purely biomechanical point of view, the coccyx and the musculature of the pelvic floor form the base of the spine and trunk and should be actively involved in all movements that support or locomote the spine. In agrarian cultures, this part of the body is still actively used in squatting to work the fields. In cultures with less furniture, the pelvic floor is used in raising and lowering to the ground. However, in industrio-technological cultures we are able to keep it passive much of the time.

The pelvic floor is the area at the base of the spine bounded by the pubic bone to the front, the sitz bones (ischial tuberosities) to the sides, and the coccyx (the tail end of the spine) to the back.

 Again sit in a vertical position, but this time let yourself slouch down. Cough, feeling your pelvic floor as you cough. Does it open up, bulge out? Cough again. Feel the extent to which this bulging can develop into an action that moves the trunk into an erect posture. Cough

again, and this time extend the sound and intensify the bulging. Find a way to fully extend your trunk into an erect posture by continuing this bulging action.

Bulging the pelvic floor a bit is one way to perform a spinal push from the pelvic floor, if those muscles were overly shortened to begin with. We might use this action in giving birth, having a bowel movement, lifting a heavy object, or in merely supporting our pelvis and trunk. A whale uses this action to propel itself forward. For humans, it is possible to stand without using this action, but standing with good posture requires it. Without employing a spinal push from the pelvic floor there is, at the very least, a subtle slouching or tense holding of the pelvis.

Psychologically this action provides a very basic sense of support. Like the push from the head, it establishes the internal space for core processing. On a physiological level, slouching in the pelvis compresses the digestive organs. Visceral emotional responses and digestive processes both require the spinal push from the tail in order to maintain the space necessary to complete their sequences with ease. For the vertically oriented human being, the push from

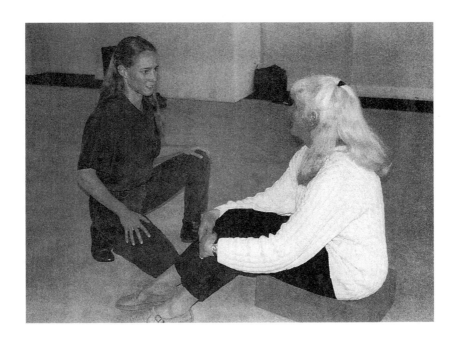

Spinal push from the pelvic floor. Notice how the woman
on the left has a strong enough push to support an erect spine
all the way through to her head. This is in contrast to the woman on the right.

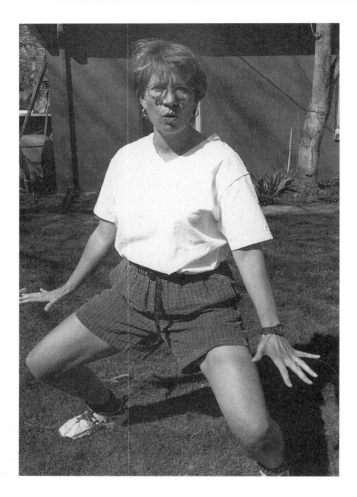

Spinal push from the pelvic floor.

the tail is very important in supporting the trunk. This support evokes a sense of empowerment, a basic feeling of confidence and capability. As infants, this action develops a sense of our inner world and brings us into contact with our inner strength. Iseman (1989) describes it as "evoking a feeling of gathering energy and root or locomotive power."

In conjunction with this action, we will look at a session with a client who was working through rape memories. Leigh reported chronic lower back pain. In this session she described an incident of encountering someone who frightened her. As she described the scenario, her voice and her stance both weakened. Specifically, Leigh's pelvis, which was normally in an extended posi-

tion, became even more pulled back. When asked to notice what she was feeling in her pelvic area, she experienced "fear and drawing back." She noticed that the fear and drawing back both emanated from the same area that chronically hurt. Her rape memories rushed in, and she began crying and gesturing away from her body with her hands. Over a period of half an hour, as emotional intensity ebbed and flowed, we generalized the protective pushing gesture she had begun with her hands. Leigh allowed this gesture to spread first into her legs and finally into her pelvic floor (perineum). She recognized this pushing of the pelvic floor as an exact reversal of the "fear and drawing back" gesture. She also experienced pushing with the pelvic floor as a way to literally "push [the rapist] out." She felt "relieved, and like I can face the world" as she transitioned into a new stance that included the spinal push with the tail. This action allowed her to complete the sequencing of her anger. It also empowered her to protect herself by pushing away rather than engaging. Leigh practiced telling people to go away; there was conviction in her voice and her stance. Overall she felt pleased with herself, as if discovering a new possibility.

Wilhelm Reich observed that, in simple organisms, plasma flows away from pain. Using the push through the pelvic floor was a way, in this case, to reverse that flow of withdrawal from the rape trauma. Often this action is important in sexual trauma and toilet training issues. Generally there is a sense of empowerment when the push from the pelvic floor is discovered physically. Again, this action was not drawn on formulaically, but arose spontaneously in relation to the rape trauma. It was introduced gesturally by the client herself as she became fearful. Since our culture is so fearful of power and sexuality, I find that most of us need to continually invite ourselves to stay alive in our pelvic floors, inviting their creative resources. We tend to underestimate the amount of power and aliveness that is possible in this area of our bodies.

HOMOLOGOUS PUSH FROM THE HANDS

This action is a coordinated push with both hands. When it sequences fully and properly, it goes all the way through the trunk, down into the pelvic floor, and through the legs into the feet. Try this.

Stand arm's length from a wall, weight evenly on both feet. Place your hands against the wall at shoulder height. Lean into your hands and let your body fall toward the wall. Now press into the wall with your hands. Feel that pressing action spread through your arms, down your trunk, and, if possible, all the way to your feet. If your feet press lightly into the floor, you can feel an isometric fullness or tautness between your hands and your feet.

The push that extends all the way from the hands to the feet is the fullest sequence of this basic neurological action, the homologous push from the upper body. Babies often use this action to slide backward on their bellies. Children (and adults) sometimes use this action gesturally to say "no," set a limit, or express anger. Adults might use this action to push away from the table, do a handstand, push an object, or keep someone from getting close.

Psychologically, proper use of this action seems to go along with the ability to be emotionally separate, to assert oneself, and to set boundaries interpersonally, specifically to say "no." When connecting to this action people describe such feelings as "taking my life into my hands," and feeling "clear and firm about my limits." Bonnie Cohen (1984) talks about this pattern: "Children who are sat early a lot do not develop full strength and action

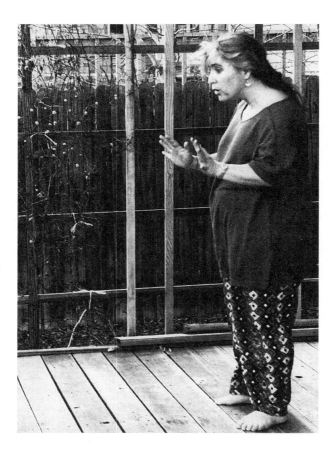

Homologous push from the hands sequencing
from the hands to the chest but not into the head or pelvis.

through their arms. Adults with this problem express feeling inadequate in acting upon their environment."

In a movement therapy group, members were working with partners exploring how close they wished to be to each other, walking toward and away from each other. Elijah, a group member, would repeatedly reach out as his partner came close to arm's length. As his partner continued to approach, he would embrace her. He reported feeling "scared. . . . I didn't want her to come any closer." This young man had a history of prolonged sexual abuse by a family member and a current history of promiscuity bordering on prostitution. In this work with his partner, Elijah initiated a homologous push from the upper by extending his arms as his partner approached. However, the action of separation became an embrace. His only experience with resolving fear was to allow the person in. He did not have an experience of setting a limit and asserting the message "Don't come any closer." We worked with his partner slowly approaching and retreating while he attended to his body and his impulses. Eventually Elijah was able to feel and follow an impulse to push with his hands against his partner's body, prohibiting her approach. At this point his eyes teared: "I don't understand. I feel confused. I mean I do understand. This is what I do, isn't it?" This was the beginning of a new insight and a new behavior for him. In the next group he received feedback from the group members about what they had seen. He clarified intellectually his understanding of his pattern of drawing threatening contacts closer to him. Elijah understood his new option, and felt vulnerable and poignant about the possibility of practicing it.

In Elijah we see an extreme case of a poorly developed homologous push from the upper. The issue of setting external boundaries is commonly expressed in relation to this action. Iseman (1989) reports an adult's experience of performing this action the way a baby does it, lying belly down and pushing with the hands to lift the head and chest and slide backward: "When I finally arrived at the top of the push, elbows extended, head supported, with a feeling of power and support throughout my whole upper torso, I quite suddenly experienced a hitherto unfamiliar feeling of self-supporting empowerment. I felt exhilarated. Then, all of a sudden, I started to feel isolated, too independent and separate, too powerful. 'If I allow myself to become grounded and supported in this position, then I won't need anyone else.'" This is almost identical to the dilemma in which Elijah found himself, defining a new style of relationship based on boundary-setting as opposed to powerlessness. The cues for pursuing this action were his initial gesture of extending the arms, and then the discrepancy between his desires and actions as he found himself embracing his partner even when he didn't want her to come any closer.

Homologous Push with the Feet

This action is a unified push of both feet. Properly sequenced, it continues up the legs, through the trunk, and out the head and hands. Many people have difficulty sequencing this action past the waist, and for most people the action gets stuck somewhere in the trunk.

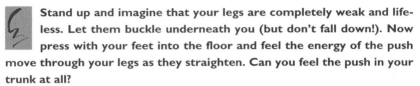 **Stand up and imagine that your legs are completely weak and lifeless. Let them buckle underneath you (but don't fall down!). Now press with your feet into the floor and feel the energy of the push move through your legs as they straighten. Can you feel the push in your trunk at all?**

If possible, find a doorway or stairwell or something overhead under which you can stand. Push up into it with the palms of your hands. (If you can't find anything, go back to the wall you used for the push from the upper.) Relax the legs again and, as you begin pressing into the floor with your feet, also begin pressing with your hands. See if the counterforce of pressing through the hands allows you to sequence the push of the feet further up into the trunk. (Don't be discouraged if this doesn't go all the way through. This is tricky, even with live facilitation and feedback.)

The homologous push from the feet is a necessary action for standing. The more fully it is sequenced, the more securely we are able to stand and the more supported the trunk is by the legs. This action is so ongoing that we take it for granted, but when we view it with a trained eye we see that it varies tremendously from person to person.

Psychologically, the degree to which we are able to sustain a homologous push from the feet seems consistent with our sense of support, stability, and the abilities to "stand on our on two feet," "take a stand," and "stick up for ourselves." People report feeling grounded and very present with this action. Since both feet are pushing and are therefore unavailable to reach to take a step, this position can have an unequivocal quality to it. This is somewhat true in all the homologous patterns. Since both limbs are doing the same thing, there is an "all or nothing" quality to these actions. The push from the feet "can have an age two stubbornness about it" (Iseman, 1989). Further development into the homolateral patterns allows greater flexibility and negotiability. Again I will illustrate this action with an extreme case.

Dorothy was a developmentally delayed client in her late forties who had led an extremely sheltered existence in her parents' home until they died. The words "extremely sheltered" hardly describe their lifestyle. Groceries were always delivered. Dorothy hardly left her home after graduating from high school. Her time was spent watching television and filling a series of notebooks with soap opera-

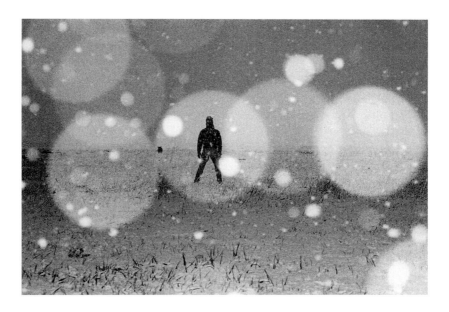

Homologous push from the feet.

like fantasies that ran on endlessly. Upon the death of her parents (which occurred within months of each other), Dorothy was tested, diagnosed as borderline retarded with general developmental delays, and placed within a group home program for the retarded. This program planned for her to begin work at a sheltered workshop, but the first obstacle was getting there. Dorothy felt she was unable to walk three blocks to the bus stop. Her ankles buckled under her continually; in standing, she rolled in on her ankles severely. In addition, her mental state was distraught about her sudden lack of support and her ability to survive. Out of all this, she rapidly entered into very depressed behavior, staying in bed whenever possible and refusing food.

The inroad to working with Dorothy was her stubbornness and her propensity toward tantrums. This seemed to be where her energy lay. She would spend movement sessions ranting and raving about how this program was killing her and how her parents would avenge her abuse if they were not dead. Though this behavior was initially overwhelming for me, it quickly developed into a way of rousing energy in positive directions, finding humor, and activating her legs. As Dorothy expressed her anger, she was encouraged to let that expression spread down into her feet. This was done by having her move with bare feet (greater sensory activation) and giving her lots of positive reinforcement for loud stamping and jumping. As her energy was drawn down into her feet during the movement sessions, she also exercised the only power to which she had access—power like that of the "terrible twos," "no" power, "I won't" power.

Outside of the sessions, Dorothy became less prone to twisting her ankles. She shed her high-heel boots and bought walking shoes, and she became more confident about her ability to walk to the bus, specifically, and to support herself in general.

This case is an interesting expression of this action, because initially Dorothy had all the psychological expressions of push—that is, standing her ground regarding staying in bed, not eating, and not walking—yet, she had nearly no physical ability to push with her feet. She could hardly stand up. The issue of support is present in nearly every way on every level here. All of us are faced with times when we wish to give up supporting ourselves. As adults this is often an ineffective way of getting what we want. Being sensitive to the energy sequencing through our legs can enable us to make more conscious choices about supporting ourselves.

HOMOLATERAL PUSH FROM THE HAND

Like the homologous push from the hands, the homolateral push from the hand sequences from the hand down through the trunk and potentially into the leg and foot. The difference between the two actions is that in this action only one hand pushes, and that push sequences down the same side of the body into the foot on the same side, rather than through the whole body into both feet. Like the homologous push, this action offers support, but with greater flexibility. The stubborn, unequivocal quality of the homologous is not present. Yet the strength of the homologous push underlies the homolateral push. Once the baby can push strongly with both hands, she begins is to support her whole upper body on one hand, reaching or playing with the other hand. This is an example of the way in which this action is used for physical support. When infants use it to locomote on their bellies, one hand pushes and it slides the body backward in an arc. Visually, this movement is lovely, and the psychological flexibility that it offers is quite apparent from the shape of the movement.

Adults often use this movement gesturally, one hand pushing out in a gesture that says, "Let's slow down," while the other hand might remain open to possibility. This is qualitatively quite different from both hands gesturing a "no," creating a firm boundary. There is often a lot of dignity present in the person who fully embodies this homolateral action, as there is the possibility of maintaining one's boundaries clearly with the pushing side while the other side is free to reach out or otherwise engage with the world. In locomoting on the floor, this movement arcs the spine, the eyes are moved in a scanning fashion. Scanning gives a sense of overview, which also might be associated with dignity or being in a good position. The rhythm of this movement as it extends from side to side has a grace to it that contrasts with the bluntness of

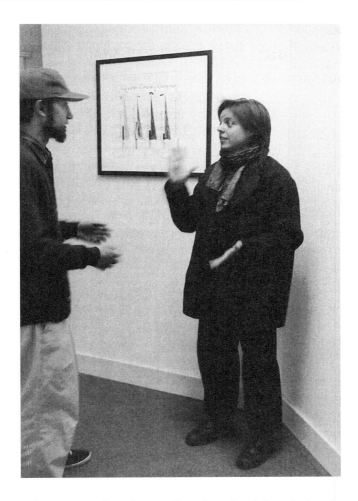

The person on the right uses a homolateral push from the hand,
which sequences into her upper spine.

the homologous. At times all of these qualities come together in a compelling
suggestion of maturity.

> **Explore this action with another person. First face each other with
> both hands up and ready to push. How does the relationship feel in
> this stance? Then take one hand down. How does it feel different to
> push with just one hand? Your other hand is free to relate however it wants.**

Developmentally, this action is not as involved in the nitty gritty of core
psychological issues as those already described. However, it is important in

relationship issues in the balancing of separation and intimacy. We will look at one case vignette that involves both this action and the next.

HOMOLATERAL PUSH FROM THE FOOT

This action involves a push from one foot that potentially sequences all the way up that side of the body and out the hand of the same side. This is the primary action used by lizards for locomotion. Like the other pushes from the lower body, it is a basic supporting action. Like the homolateral push with the hand, this action offers more maneuverability than the homologous. One foot is able to sufficiently push to support the rest of the body. The other foot is thereby free to step, to advance or retreat. The uncompromising stance of the homologous matures; there are more choices available. One is confident enough of one's support that one can move out from it to explore surrounding territory.

To experience this action, begin with the homologous push with the feet. Take a stance with both feet evenly planted. Release your weight into them and feel solid in this position. Notice your state of mind. How does this posture affect it? Then shift your weight onto one foot. See if you can feel as fully supported on one foot as you did on two. Spend a moment or two in this position. Look around yourself from this place. Is there any difference in your state of mind? Does the world appear any different?

To explore both of the homolateral pushes, we can look at the dilemma in which one woman found herself. Liza had spent most of her life "following the straight and narrow." As she matured, she found herself exploring a more adventurous side of herself, but this seemed to get her in trouble. She got confused. She didn't know "which end was up." She got mixed up in uncomfortable relationships and she had to "pull herself back together" all the more as a result. In talking, she illustrated the "together" mode in a very homologous fashion; square on both feet, lots of push, no receptivity. Liza realized that she couldn't let anybody or any possibilities in within this stance. It wasn't any fun, but it was safe. On the other hand, it was lots of fun to just let go into adventure. She did this by letting go of any push and flowing gleefully hither and thither. But since this strategy wasn't safe, it did not work for her either. So Liza's options were homologous push with both hands with its very strong boundaries (I can't let anyone in) coupled with homologous push with both feet with its strong support (but no flexibility), or letting go of all boundaries and support. The quest for the homolateral was expressed in her desire to meld the two, but it was not in her current repertoire of energetic possibilities. However, her movement was integrated enough, and she was emotionally well-balanced enough that it was possible to simply introduce the homolateral option. This was done with the upper and lower bodies simultaneously, feeling the push from one hand and one foot meet

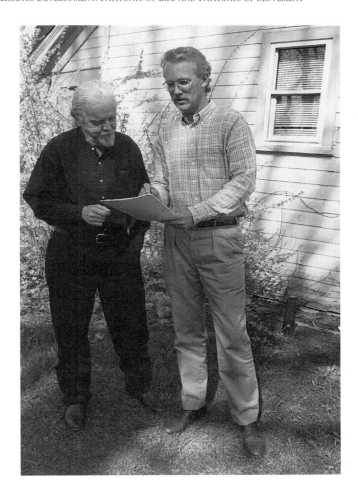

Homolateral push from the foot. The man on the right is pushing
with just his right foot, while the man on the
left has a more homologous push.

*as they filled one side. What this created for her was a sense of the midline of her
body. It amazed her to have two sides with two different feelings. The pushing side
felt "strong and clear," and the other side felt "open, less-formed." Liza practiced relating to others this way, and found herself more able to "come and go." When there
was a sense of threat or conflict, she could explore that without solidifying her homologous fortress. When there was a sense of invitation, she could be open to this
without diving in. What the homolateral organization offered Liza was a way to unify
two qualities that she already understood.*

SPINAL REACH FROM THE HEAD

Having explored pushes from all the endpoints, we now turn to the reaching actions.

 With your trunk in a vertical but collapsed position, close your eyes. Imagine an object dangling over your head. Feel the skin of your scalp. Let it wake up, becoming curious about the object overhead. As if searching through the air to find it, let the top of your head reach up into space. As your head reaches higher and higher, feel it draw your trunk into an upright position. Feel the lightness of your trunk that the reach creates.

The reach of the head is closely linked with alertness. The senses of the head reaching out to gather information create a movement that draws the whole spine into space. The quintessential display of this is when a long-necked animal, such as a deer, smells something. As if a string were attached to its nose, the deer's head is drawn down and forward in the direction of the smell.

Psychologically the reach of the head engages one with the outside world. The senses become alert. This may be attended by qualities of inquisitiveness and curiosity, if there is adequate support. On the other hand, without adequate support there might be feelings of lightheadedness or disorientation. Often this action is associated with intellect because of the involvement of the head and brain. The following example illustrates this association.

Jamie was a college student who was labeled learning-disabled as a child. As an adult, he struggled to read, think, write, and understand his world conceptually. Though these were very awkward processes for him, he focused tremendous energy in that direction. His posture looked as if someone had pressed down on his head, pushing it down between his shoulders and causing him to hunch in his thoracic spine. His movement was very muscular, with a great deal of push. His thinking reflected this. Jamie labored his way through abstractions; in attempting to grasp a new concept, his eyes clouded and his forehead constricted. He discovered pushing with his head through imitation, and he delighted in it, playfully nuzzling into the floor. This seemed to be easily accessible and relieved the congestion in his head while he did it, but the congested feeling returned when he stopped pushing. Jamie carried a great deal of self-criticism regarding his intellectual abilities. This self-criticism and frustration was paired with the congested feeling in his head. There was no possibility of simply relaxing this; it needed to be redirected. In a classroom situation, Jamie learned the spinal reach of the head. In a hands-and-knees position, he allowed his head to be lightly stimulated on top and gently drawn out. Out of this, he began reaching with his head to crawl. He had been born in a breech position; this action of reaching through the head therefore felt like a com-

pletely foreign possibility. There is no way to describe the quality of the shift that occurred as he explored this new action. Jamie was amazed and confused. There was a relaxation and a lifting of tension in the whole room. Fellow students described it as a magical change. He continued to explore this action, receiving verbal and tactile feedback both within this class and in ensuing classes. His posture changed. The quality of his writing changed. There was less concrete repetition, and less asking questions for others to answer. This shift made room for independent exploration.

The pattern of retracting the head is commonly paired with a sense of intellectual inadequacy. It is also linked with sensory withdrawal, and, in these cases, may or may not have connection to the intellect. Like the push of the head, it is commonly related to birthing experiences, particularly the phase of actual delivery. In general, it is common to have learned to limit one's innate curiosity about the world by limiting the energy of reach in one's head. In turn, this energetic limitation restricts us in many ways.

SPINAL REACH FROM THE PELVIC FLOOR

Like all the reaches, the initiation of this action requires an awakening of the sense perceptions in the tissue of the reaching endpoint. Culturally we are very uncomfortable with this action because we associate sensory wakefulness in the pelvic floor with sexual arousal. This is unfortunate, as there is a great deal more possibility in this action than just sexuality. A reach of the tail can be used to adjust our center of gravity over uneven terrain or under a moving trunk. Being sensitive and actively responsive in the pelvic floor is one skill that distinguishes those we call "naturally gifted" movers.

Close your eyes and take a wide stance with your feet apart. Imagine that you have quite a long tail, so long that you can actually sweep the ground with it. Let yourself feel your tail curling and uncurling, moving through space to explore what you cannot see. Let this movement gently shift your trunk in different directions: forward, backward, and to the sides. As you begin to feel the end of your spine and your pelvic floor awakening, try standing on one foot. Use your hands to support you as needed. Give your tail more permission to reach and explore space. Feel the quality of moving your trunk when your pelvic floor is initiating.

Psychologically, this is a very fruitional action. To be free to explore in the pelvic floor requires a well-established sense of support. One needs to trust one's ground well enough to play with it. It also seems to draw on earthy intelligence, not just in garnering support but in actually being sensitive to the earthy, primitive world in a fuller way. The image of the divining rod perfectly describes this action as a way of testing the elemental qualities of what lies

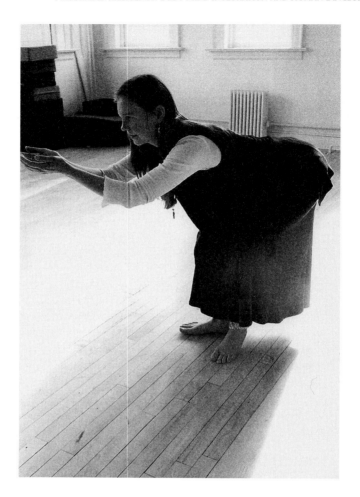

Spinal reach from the pelvic floor, which sequences
through the spine into the lower thoracic.

below. Initially, as the emotions of sexual traumas, anger, or toilet training
complexes are released in the pelvic floor, the push is very active. Slowly, as
this push is established and confidence develops, the reach can begin to come
into play. In my experience, this action often arises fleetingly at first, perhaps
following a release in the pelvic area that resolves as a moment of openness.
Exploring this action after such a glimpse often renews creativity or brings a
new ability to initiate sexually. Developmentally, this action is quite advanced and allows the mover to explore new possibilities without external
support.

Claude was a sculptor whose wife was considering leaving him. He felt extremely vexed by her dissatisfaction. His face would scowl, his hands would make fists, and he'd draw his head down. He couldn't understand what the problem was. They had a good life. Their children were grown. They'd always been happy. Things were fine. His wife had suggested that they go into therapy to help understand each other. She felt bored and uninspired by their relationship. She felt that it was stagnant at a time when she wanted growth. She felt that all his creative energy went into his art and that none went toward their relationship.

When Claude talked about his work, his head would reach with exquisite delicacy. He entered a world of wonder. You could almost see the world around him begin to sparkle and glow. His wife said, "That's what I want. That's the kind of attention I want you to bring to our relationship." Claude returned to his scowl. When I asked Claude about their early relationship, he described it as tremendously passionate. He felt that sort of driving lust was no longer possible at their age, and furthermore that his wife rejected him when he approached her with that energy. As he moved his body, there was much more quality of push around this topic. I talked to him about his bodily experience of being in his studio, sculpting. With direction, he became aware of the magical, delicate quality of reach that he was using. I asked him to imagine that he had another head at the bottom of his trunk that could look out at the world in a similar way as the head on top. Because he was such an imaginative person, this quirky image worked for him. The quality of reach permeated his trunk and his whole being altogether. He looked at his wife, as if for the first time. The room had a quality like waking up from a dream. This moment became a template from which they reconstructed their relationship, to include the spinal reach from the pelvic floor.

HOMOLOGOUS REACH FROM THE HANDS

One of the most poignant images for this action is that of a small child reaching up to an adult. Both arms are extended, the head is also reaching, and there is a sense of complete longing, "Uppie, uppie." This action is a reach of both hands. The more awake the skin of the palms is, the stronger the initiation. The sequence can move through the arms and continue down the full length of the body. The completion of this action might result in a dive or a slide into base. This action is the beginning of an embrace. It may also be a beseechment to the heavens. Infants often use it in the sitting position; they see an object and both hands reach toward it, pulling the body along until they fall, and, usually, land on the object of desire. This happens before they develop the ability to reach with one hand and maintain their position.

Psychologically with this action we encounter again the "full-out" quality of the homologous. In this case, it is a full-out reach. This is an expression of whole-hearted desire. "All of me wants that," with no reservations. The image of a prophet in the desert, crying out to his god, comes to mind, or a farmer welcoming the rain, or the coming together of two loved ones. The difficulty for adults seems to be in exposing oneself to potential disappointment, or purely exposing one's heart, period. Without support, this reach can become a fall, like the infant's fall toward the toy. With support, as adults we can extend ourselves to the world, tolerating both the exposure and the possibility of our desire being unrequited.

 In a joint family therapy group, Nathan was discussing his relationship with his wife. This man described his sexual advances toward her using words like "enthusiastic" and "grab." The difficulty he experienced was that he often

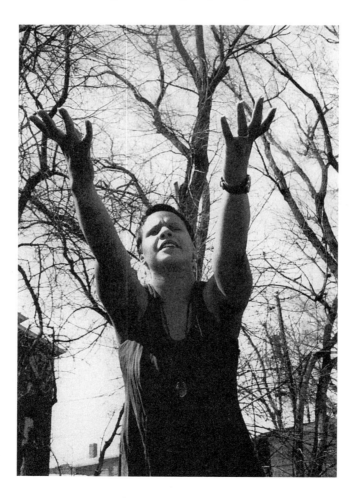

Homologous reach from the hands.

overwhelmed her, and she retreated. He felt rebuffed. "I was just reaching out to her," he told us. As he demonstrated with a group member, we saw that there was in fact very little "reaching out" involved. Instead Nathan seemed to be propelling himself toward her. The image of pouncing seemed apt. A pounce is initiated more from a push from the lower body than from a reach from the upper body. As a group we played with reaching movements of the hands. The atmosphere in the room became more sensitive and vulnerable. We experimented with standing in place but reaching toward a partner with both hands. Members of the group took turns viewing each other. They observed that people varied in how much they were actually reaching out energetically. They described this action as creating a feeling of openheartedness and vulnerability. The group observed that the men in this group were less able to reach fully with both hands than the women. A discussion ensued in which the men revealed feeling that they were expected not to be vulnerable in this way, but rather to take instead of reach. Nathan developed awareness of his reluctance to be vulnerable with his wife.

In general, this is an action that most adults leave by the wayside as they leave childhood. It remains in adulthood only in subtle, gestural remnants. Often when people are ready for it emotionally, they are surprised to find that they enjoy the blatant enthusiasm it holds.

HOMOLOGOUS REACH FROM THE FEET

This action is one that we rarely get to perform fully, simply because our legs are usually supporting us. Children do this action when sliding off a bed or down the stairs feet first. Both feet are reaching and that pulls the body along; adults may employ it in coming out of a handstand or reaching to the ground from a tree branch. Though its full execution is rare, the homologous reach from the feet is an important action energetically. It is the ability to release energy out both legs and feet.

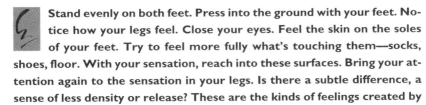 **Stand evenly on both feet. Press into the ground with your feet. Notice how your legs feel. Close your eyes. Feel the skin on the soles of your feet. Try to feel more fully what's touching them—socks, shoes, floor. With your sensation, reach into these surfaces. Bring your attention again to the sensation in your legs. Is there a subtle difference, a sense of less density or release? These are the kinds of feelings created by reaching, an action which energetically allows us to move out.**

This action is difficult to contact because we do it so infrequently. It can also be imagined by reaching with the hands and then transferring that feeling into the legs. Just like the other reaches, it is necessary for the skin to be awake. Touch is a good way to stimulate the sensory nerves.

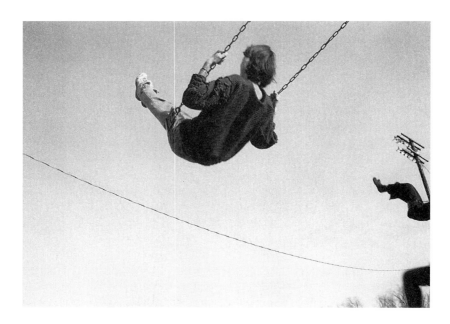

Homologous reach from the feet sequencing into the front of the pelvis.

With bare feet, rub and touch the soles of your feet to wake them up. Lay down with your feet close to, but not touching, an object on the floor. Without looking, reach feet first to contact and then to explore the object.

The psychological component implicit in reaching from both feet is often subtle. As with all reaching movements, there is the element of engaging, going out to the world. Basic energetic health seems to require input and output flowing regularly through all the avenues of the body. The feet need to release and give up their supporting role periodically. This seems to evoke playful qualities and mitigate feelings of "heaviness" about one's responsibilities.

Jeanine, a client with a chronic eating disorder, engaged in a movement therapy group as part of an inpatient treatment program in a hospital. Jeanine was extremely controlled and rigid. She suffered from chronic constipation that was now exacerbated by being on a hospital-controlled diet. In complaining of this, she was led to memories of her parents' attitudes toward her toilet training. They were full of pride that she accomplished it so quickly and easily. Jeanine expressed bitterness toward them, and, as she did so, began squirming in her legs. A group member noticed this and began to play with her around this movement, grab-

bing her legs. Jeanine directed her partner to use firm pressure. She began to struggle, and her partner resisted her struggle, matching her efforts. This continued for a long time, and then the struggle slowly died down. Although the partner continued to respond to the movements of Jeanine's legs with touch, the quality became more one of caressing. Jeanine's movements began to take on a reaching, luxurious quality. Jeanine expressed pleasure and relaxation in her face. Afterward, she shared that she had liked the struggle, and she felt very relaxed now.

In conjunction with toilet training, and likely in response to the whole family atmosphere, Jeanine had restricted any release in her lower body. There was literally a drawing up and tightening of the musculature in her legs and pelvis. Through exaggerating this, she was able to release it and allow a reach to happen. This brought her into a nurturing relationship with another, which was unusual for her.

The homologous reach from the feet usually brings with it some sense of relief. For Jeanine it was an initial release of the restriction maintained in her whole lower body. Out of this she may eventually be able to release her pelvic floor, which was definitely the seed of the whole pattern. However, that was too threatening for her to approach at the time. To allow the legs to reach first was an initial thaw.

Our feet and legs serve us in carrying our weight so much of the time that it is rare that they are offered the chance to play, to initiate their own explorations. Such explorations might open up unexpected energy and new options.

CONTRALATERAL REACH FROM THE HAND

This action is the main initiative in crawling on hands and knees (technically known as creeping). In creeping, one hand reaches out and pulls diagonally across the body, drawing the opposite knee forward. However, without the support of all the other earlier actions, this movement would not be possible. The ability of the limbs to push, individually and in a coordinated manner, keeps the body supported upon hands and knees. The spinal connection from head to tail, established by a continuous dialogue of pushing and reaching from end to end, maintains the internal integrity of the trunk. All of this frees the hand to reach out and draw the body along with it.

Adults use this pattern to organize a large number of movements, anything from shaking hands to writing. It is visible when, from a stationary standing position, one reaches a hand toward an object. If the object is far enough away, this reach of the hand pulls diagonally across the body and draws the opposite leg into taking a step. Whenever and however an adult uses this movement, it is being supported by the earlier, more primitive movements.

When there is difficulty in executing a contralateral movement, generally it is due to a weakness in one of the earlier patterns.

Psychologically, the contralateral reach from the hand is an integration of the support and engagement derived from the earlier actions. It is the ability to reach out while maintaining internal support and interpersonal boundaries. This is different from diving in or giving up one's ground in order to make contact. Rather, it is a level of extending out to the world in which we are free to express and interact while staying grounded in our own being. Often the attempt to reach out in this mature and balanced fashion is made difficult because one of the underlying stages is not been adequately developed. However, there is a stage of both physical and psychological development in which the individual is ready to take on this action. This was true in the following case.

 Gregg was a middle-aged man with a disturbing family history, a barely normal intelligence level, and some minimal signs of organic brain damage possibly associated with birth and other early childhood traumas. Gregg had been institutionalized since his adolescence and was currently in a community treatment program for retarded and handicapped adults. He had been a part of this program for ten years, since the time of its inception. He was quite comfortable in it and had received consistent emotional counseling, tutoring, and job training. He had cultivated friendships and leisure activities that he enjoyed. He was beginning to work outside of the system, and this was where his current difficulties lay. In the past, as soon as he had accomplished a goal, there was an obvious next step on which to focus. This time the focus remained on his success and maturation. This was emotionally very threatening to him, and he began to sabotage himself. Each time he received good feedback at a new job site he would stop showing up for work. This was in contrast to his reliable attendance at sheltered workshop and job training.

In an individual therapy session, Gregg was discussing the various jobs he had "screwed up" recently. He was asked to place each job at a different spot in the room. He sat in the middle of the floor and positioned the jobs at various points on the edge of the room. Concentrating on one, he would reach toward the spot with one hand and that would begin to pull his body toward it in a crawl. But at the very end of that hand's reach, he would draw back, jamming his wrist and elbow joints and falling back on his buttocks. There was no lack of support inhibiting his reaching the spot; it was purely a reversal or pulling back of the reach. Gregg repeated this pattern again and again, focusing on each spot in turn. He seemed to enjoy the ritualistic quality of frustration. This was a perfect physical enactment of the process he had been involved in. Though he generally thought in concrete terms, the symbolism being created here was vivid enough for him to relate to it. He was grinning, continuing his ritual and saying, "This is it. This is it." I began taking his arm and compressing it back into his body as he reached out. This was replicating and taking over his re-

traction in the middle of the reach. There was a moment of locking gazes and then a play began of his pulling back and pushing into my grip. I started to repeat, "Oh no, you don't. . . oh no, you don't," in the same rhythm he had been using. As we played, I began to allow his arm to slide through my grasp as it reached. There was still a rhythm of his reaching and then my compressing, but, as I took over, he stopped retracting. Slowly I allowed the intervals to become longer until finally he reached all the way to the floor, completing the crawling step. There was a moment of surprise and stillness. I said, "Keep going." Gregg reached all the way through and began crawling around the room. As he passed through a job spot I would name it, "the drugstore. . .the florist," and so forth. In this way the game completed itself. We did not discuss the implications of this "game" because that would have been meaningless to his concrete style of thought. Nevertheless, there was a feeling of import and intimacy as we closed the session. Outside the sessions, there were several shifts. Behaviorally, he stopped arguing with the feedback that he was sabotaging himself; his support staff reported he was more able to "hear" this feedback. We continued to play crawling and reaching games for the next few sessions. His pattern of sabotaging seemed to wear down, and he eventually settled into a job.

This case is an example of a difficulty lying in a contralateral reach itself rather than in an underlying action. In this case, the contralateral reach was right on the cutting edge of Gregg's development. This phase is analogous to a toddler who has grown beyond either totally rejecting an activity or hurling himself headlong into it. At this point there may be a more hesitant approach and an attentive parent might say, "Come on, you can do it." Slowly the toddler reaches out.

The contralateral reaches represent an integration of all our means of giving and receiving from the world. Clearing up any issues at this level can be fruitional to an individual's development.

CONTRALATERAL REACH FROM THE FOOT

This action is a reach from one foot that sequences across the body and draws the opposing arm into movement. It is the basic initiator of walking. As with the contralateral reach from the hand, the support and integration of the earlier patterns allows this initiation to complete itself. While it is quite common to walk without this reach, its presence brings a sense of lightness, ease, and smoothness.

This is true psychologically as well. Like the contralateral reach from the hand, the contralateral reach from the foot signifies a certain level of maturation. It is the ability to reach out with one foot, either to explore a step in that direction or to make contact. It signifies an ability to reach while maintaining a grounded sense of one's position and boundaries. On the most literal level, it is taking a step *without* making a blind leap, and *with* one's sense of self intact. Openness and confidence to go forward are the psychological qualities that generally accompany this energetic flow outward through one leg and foot.

Cecilly had become competitive athletically at a very early age. As a promising figure skater, she was pushed to practice everyday after school, effectively cutting out any time for play. She worked her legs to the point of permanently deforming them before she chose to discontinue the sport. As a young adult she began to realize that she had never learned to recognize and follow her own impulses and had consistently been a "good girl." Psychologically she felt numb;

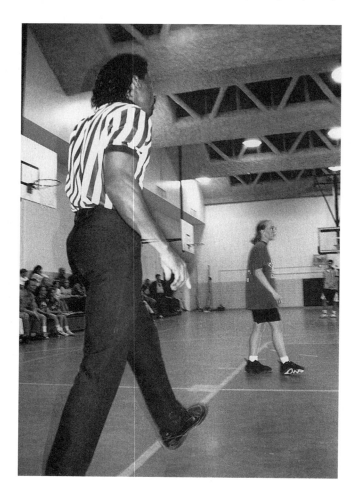

Contralateral reach from the foot.

when she checked in with her body, she discovered that her legs had the least amount of sensation. Her legs had a lot of muscular build up, and the tissue was very fatty and somewhat lifeless.

Under direction, Cecilly began to spend time focusing on her legs. At first the time felt flat and unproductive. Still, I directed her to continue to focus on the sensations in her legs and any impulses to move, and to follow these impulses as fully as possible. Slowly she began to find more activity arising during her sessions. When she shared her progress, I asked if I could touch her legs. This began a process in which I encouraged her to let her legs freely respond to my touch. She pushed and pushed and pushed against my hands with the soles of her feet. Finally exhausted, she rested. I kept my hands on the soles of her feet and, after a few moments, she began to explore my hands with her feet. She began touching my hand with one leg extended and drawing the opposite foot up, sliding it against the calf and leg of the other foot. She repeated this rhythmically, a kind of stepping gesture. Her breath relaxed into deep sighs. This felt like the first time in such a long while that she had released the energy through her legs. She described them as feeling "tingly" and "very different." Cecilly said she liked feeling one leg with the other foot because then they felt like different parts.

Somehow, in the process of repressing her own physical and emotional needs to please adults (family and coaches), Cecilly had not only bound her own energy in her legs but she had unified them. Energetically, this was a homologous state in which both legs acted as a single unit. She had been making efforts behaviorally to differentiate and become more independent. This movement process allowed that shift to occur on a physical and energetic level. Generally that allowed the behavioral shifts to deepen into greater integrity and spontaneity.

Relational Aspects of Motor Development

Each of these movements connects us to our environment in a unique way. As we yield, push, reach, grasp, and pull, we are establishing our relationship to the physical world and to the people around us. By working these basic neurological actions, we can address some of our patterns of relationship. Do I tend to push in response to new situations? Do I always yield in the face of conflict? Am I able to fully reach toward intimacy?

We can also observe how our bodies manifest these overall patterns. How do I try to grasp what I want? What endpoint or endpoints tend to embody this action for me? Where does the push to assert myself get stuck in my body? Where does it collapse?

A special branch of psychoanalysis called *object relations* explores the patterns that are set up in our first relationships with our mother and other pri-

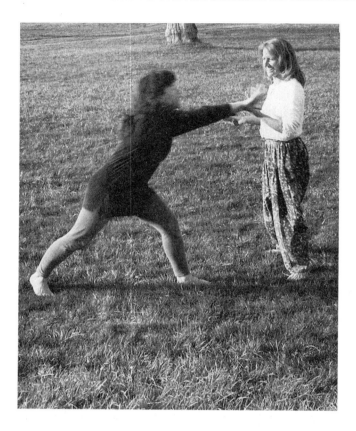

Interacting with reach and push.

mary caregivers. Object relations recognizes the impact that these early templates have on our entire life. These relational patterns are mirrored in our early motor development. As we learn to push and reach in the physical world, we are learning to interact in the interpersonal world. Thus, the two processes are closely interrelated and in some ways inseparable. These actions give us a very concrete way of working with and changing our basic patterns of relationship.

Energetic Development

Energetic development is the development of our ability to sequence energy through the body in new ways. By attending to the issues in our lives and observing the energetic shifts that occur in response to them, we can gain in-

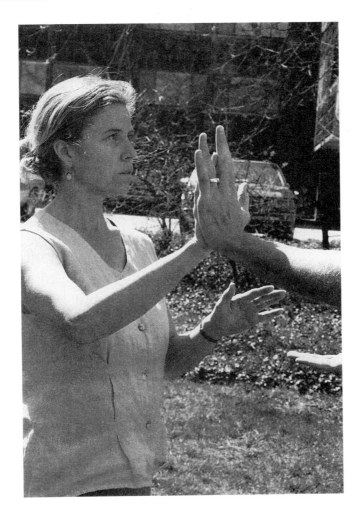

sight into the question of which developmental actions to invite or redirect. Supporting ourselves to develop is a crucial step toward embracing the possibility of growing throughout our life-span. This can occur in working with oneself in the practice of natural movement, or in the course of one's daily life, or it can occur in the process of working with others educationally or therapeutically.

In my work, the human potential for development sometimes appears to be so strong and central to our basic nature, that neglecting our development seems to violate our basic health. Thus the maxim, "If we are not growing, we are stagnating." Accepting a developmental perspective in one's life creates both great freedom and great responsibility. The freedom arises from the fact that there is always room to grow. There is always the possibility for change. The responsibility lies in the fact that we need to steward our own development; that is, we need to observe and support ourselves to make each next necessary step. A developmental perspective holds a beautiful view of human life as continual unfoldment, a process of surprise and discovery without a final stopping point. There is always another step to take. There is no longer either refuge or prison in the belief that "This is just who I am."

While a developmental perspective acknowledges that there are basic enduring qualities to each person, these qualities become more of a question than a given, and there is usually still plenty of room to move within them. For example, I might wonder how much of my emotional sensitivity is innate to me? How much of it is learned? How much of it is serving me and those around me? To what extent is my sensitivity creating obstacles? Developmentally, I might intend to cultivate the aspects of my sensitivity that best serve me while processing and completing with the aspects that are creating obstacles.

Working with the endpoints and the pathways of the developmental actions can provide a physical and energetic ground for these developmental intentions. For example, in feeling and thinking about my questions regarding sensitivity and also in observing myself at times when I feel particularly sensitive, I can observe physical and energetic patterns. When my sensitivity is serving me, I feel very grounded in my lower body. When my sensitivity is not serving me, I feel overstimulated in my upper body and less inhabited in my lower body. My upper body experiences many sensations that do not fully sequence out. Therefore, I know that, for my sensitivity to mature, I need to become more grounded in my lower body and more expressive with my upper body.

Energetic development works closely with the body-mind integration principle of sequencing. By attending to the sequencing in our bodies we can develop new ways to give and receive from the world. When energy is moving down a pathway in a radically new way, it can literally feel like growing a new limb.

Choose an area in your life in which you sense yourself trying to grow and mature. Think about it and feel your bodily responses. As you become clear about how your body responds to this issue, you will notice particular sensations that happen in particular areas. Attend to those sensations more fully. Notice if the sensations are moving toward an endpoint. (If they are not moving toward one endpoint, take a guess which

endpoint they might tend to move toward given more permission.) Wake that endpoint up. Use your breath and voice and whole body in natural movement to feel the sequencing between that endpoint and the area of sensation. (Feel free to experiment with other endpoints as needed.) As the internal movements sequence out into your endpoint, what action do you perform? Do you yield, push, reach, grasp, pull, or some combination of all of these? Complete your movement time with yourself and come back to your thoughts about this issue. Do you have a new perspective on the issue? What have you learned? Do you understand the significance of the particular developmental action(s) you ended up doing? Do you see a pathway for experimenting with bringing this action into your life more? This is energetic development.

Often we have an entirely new understanding of an issue after engaging in a process like this. We discover what energetic development needs to take place in order to resolve our dilemma. We very literally understand that we need to learn to yield, push, reach, grasp, or pull in this situation in order to move through it successfully.

To illustrate, Marcus, a competent psychotherapist was seeking supervision regarding setting limits with a particular client. While Marcus was generally able to do this, he was encountering difficulties with this particular person. In exploring this relationship he discovered a pattern of constricting his genitals and small intestine. He also twisted himself to one side as he constricted. He looked powerless, almost coquettish, as he did this. Having worked with this pattern previously he recognized it as a way he had sought favor from his father as a child. He realized that, with certain people, he returned to this strategy. In allowing himself to breathe and move with these sensations and gestures and his insights, he found a strong push through his pelvic floor, most notably, but in his other endpoints as well. He resolved that he would be more conscious about supporting himself with this client. He had a concrete direction that he could experiment with behaviorally. Next time Marcus worked with that client, he would push with his pelvic floor.

This example illustrates that although Marcus had resolved the developmental stage of self-sufficiency cognitively, he had not resolved it energetically. Working with energetic development often allows us to access developmental issues that we can't think our way through. Furthermore, energetic development offers us concrete behavioral directions with which to experiment, such as Marcus' resolve to push with his pelvic floor next time he saw his client.

Personal Inquiry and Exploration

Observe animals and babies to see clearly sequenced versions of these actions. Contrast this with the truncated versions of these actions that we see in adults. A truncated action does not sequence all the way through the body.

After doing the exercises that evoke each action, ask yourself, how do I use (or not use) this action in my life? When do I get stuck in my ability to sequence it through my body? How does this happen on a body level? What kind of response do I get from the world when I truncate this action? When might I use it more creatively?

Write about your relationship to yield, push, reach, grasp, and pull. What do these words mean to you? When is it good or bad to do these actions?

Observe others. Can you see individual actions that are important to them or missing from their repertoire? Can you see overall preferences or avoidances of the general categories of yield, push, reach, grasp, or pull? Can you see the effect that these preferences or avoidances have on their lives?

CHAPTER 5

The Major Body Systems: Diversity, Dialogue, and Community

The thin red jellies within you or within me, the bones and the marrow in the bones, The exquisite realization of health; O I say these are not the parts and gems of the body only, but of the soul, O I say now these are the soul!

Walt Whitman

WE HAVE A RICH AND VARIED LANDSCAPE OF TERRAIN AND WATERWAYS WITHIN US. INSIDE A HUMAN BEING LIVE ALL MANNER OF MOVING TISSUE AND WORKING SYSTEMS, BATHED BY FLUIDS OF MANY VARIETIES. THE INTRICACY AND INTELLIGENCE CONTAINED WITHIN OUR ANATOMY AND PHYSIOLOGY IS BOTH EXTRAORDINARILY BEAUTIFUL AND EFFECTIVE. YET, WE ARE SO DIVORCED FROM THE MIRACLES INSIDE US.

❀ ❀ ❀

We go through our day feeling a familiar range of limited sensations and functioning in habitual modes. But, for most of us, these are only a fraction of the possibilities within. To live fully, we go beyond our accustomed way of living in our bodies and begin to explore the full range of possibilities available to us as human animals. The basic neurological actions provide a framework of *pathways* through which energy circulates within the body. Studying the major body systems provides a sense of the *vehicles* along which this energy circulates.

While we all need our body systems to perform their basic physiological functions, a great deal of creative variety is possible beyond this baseline. For example, we vary as to how fluidly the systems coordinate functions between themselves. There is also great variety in how we organize leadership and responsiveness within this group of systems. We vary as to how we prioritize activities within ourselves and transition from one activity to another.

There is also tremendous variation in how much we attend to each system. Our attention to the various aspects of our internal and external experience coordinates our behavior. Just like the conductor of a symphony, our attention can emphasize and diminish different aspects of our bodily functioning. Consciousness of this process allows us to evolve with more intentionality. On the other hand, ignoring our bodily processes can lead to disintegration or stagnation. It is impossible to exactly specify the effects of our attentive process. However, we can feel subtle shifts of attention within ourselves and observe them in others, and we can expand our repertoire. To do this, we need to study and experience the body systems.

Much of my own study of the body systems comes from the perspective of Body-Mind Centering; however, there are other approaches to experiential anatomy. Every approach tends to focus on different elements of the body and to emphasize different aspects of experience. Each individual has their own areas of interest and unique experience of different parts of the body. I have been informed by the experiences of other teachers, the experiences of my students, as well as my own explorations.

I bring a uniquely psychological point of view to experiential anatomy. Central to this perspective is the recognition that every aspect of a biological entity has *motivation*. In humans, our rudimentary motivations blossom into emotional qualities or tones which in turn blend into full-blown emotions. Thus in exploring the body with an openness to emotion, we learn more about the personal aspects of the sensation. It is possible to explore sensation from a very objective point of view. This is akin to studying the demographics of a person's life versus hearing their story.

Studying the resources, perceptions, and emotional tone of the body systems greatly enhances our ability to be inclusive of all parts of ourselves. It is akin to learning about the different types of wildflowers in your ecosystem, or a government learning of all the various peoples in its domain. Out of this inclusivity, we are naturally drawn toward dialogue. When we are respectfully aware of our inner constituency, we are conscious of the different voices within us. We can allow those voices to dialogue in a manner that can further the whole. Issues, memories, resources, energy, and positions that were previously unconscious, half-conscious, or inarticulate can emerge with greater clarity. This is the path of development.

Furthermore, this process feeds back into the process of embodied relationship. By discovering the community within ourselves and learning to negotiate and dialogue within it, we further our ability to create dialogue and form community outside ourselves. This happens primarily in two ways. First of all, we deeply learn and experience the basic skills of negotiation and dialogue when we do it within ourselves. Through this process we get firsthand a sense of the benefits of cooperative community. Secondly, we clear our internal issues that perpetuate conflict and devalue diversity. This frees us up to dialogue with the outside world much more effectively.

The format for this chapter will be individual discussions of the major body systems, including physical and psychological characteristics and case vignettes. For the purposes of introducing this way of thinking, we will look at only the broadest divisions. However, the level of detail possible with this approach is nearly infinite. There are 256 different types of cells in the body; these group together to form various kinds of tissues which again group together to create functional systems. Each of these groupings has an individual and distinct identity, complete with unique experiences and possibilities.

One limitation of this approach is the danger of stereotyping the unique qualities of each tissue or fluid. While a given tissue or fluid may have particular qualities and modes of expression that are quite striking, there may be quieter tendencies that are not easily generalized. In addition, each of us is unique in how we use a particular tissue or fluid within us. As each of these major systems is presented, the reader is asked to remember that this is only one view. Even more so with the body systems than with the basic neurological actions, the intricate possibilities of interrelationship make rigid definitions useless.

Another limitation to keep in mind is that the systems are harder to write about than the actions discussed in the previous chapter. The actions function basically in the nervous system—the system of language—and are shape-oriented. Both of these qualities make them more accessible through the written word than the qualitative movements of the tissues and fluids. Careful reading, repetition of the exercises, and ongoing contemplation of your sensations should support greater understanding.

Despite these limitations, you will find it tremendously helpful to begin to get acquainted with these various members of our internal community. As you explore these systems, some will be very familiar—they will feel like "home." These may be the systems you innately attend to. We all have natural leaders within our communities. These are the body systems that initiate and inform much of your activity. We are also taught particular preferences by our families and culture. Learning about the qualities of your leading systems can enhance your organization.

On the other hand, some systems may feel very foreign. Again this might be innate or it might be learned. In either case, there is often great benefit in becoming more familiar with the parts of us that are most quiet or repressed. We may discover unknown resources or the root of particular obstacles.

I encourage you to experiment with this material and let these explorations unfold over time. Ongoing contemplation can offer both flashes of insight and a slowly growing sense of community and wholeness. Keep in mind also that this chapter introduces only the largest contingencies. Once you forge a relationship to each of the major systems, you may go on to break them down into many constituent parts and explore the parts in a similar manner.

The systems presented here are chosen because of their accessibility. In experiential anatomy, there is a general hierarchy ranging from that which is generally easier to access to that which is more difficult. By *access*, I mean feel, inhabit, and occupy. Within any system or tissue type, there is a nearly infinite ability to experience finer and finer levels of detail. For example, our ability to experience our brain as a whole is a precursor to our ability to differentiate the cerebellum from the frontal lobes of the cerebrum.

In another dimension, some tissue types are quieter than others; for example, the ligaments are quieter than the muscles. By *quieter*, I mean that the sensations are more subtle, less intense. It is generally easier to begin with systems or tissues that have louder sensations. For this reason, I have not included many connective tissues in this initial introduction. As your ability to listen to your body develops, your ability to make fine discriminations and to hear "quieter" signals increases.

Beyond the ability to feel different aspects of our anatomy comes the skill of initiating activity from these different aspects. *Initiating* is the action of taking leadership. It could mean beginning an action. It could mean guiding or shaping an action begun by some other part. On an experiential level, initiating feels more active and involved than just sensing or feeling. Your ability to initiate from different parts of your body will develop over time with attention and practice.

A final note before we begin examining particular systems. My intention with this chapter is to introduce the reader to a direct experience of his or her own tissues and fluids. Everyday words make us feel more at home than more technical anatomical terms. It is easier to experience skin, when you call it "skin," than when you call it the integumentary system. Therefore, whenever a common name exists, I will use that over the formal anatomical term. In some areas, this is not possible; for example, in the endocrine system, to just say "glands" confuses exocrine and endocrine glands. These are areas where we need to go further linguistically so that we can communicate our experiences as directly as possible.

Organs

Let's begin at our core, our internal, visceral organs. If the body is our home, the organs—or viscera—are the hearth, the very center of our home. The visceral organs include our respiratory system, heart, digestive system, spleen,

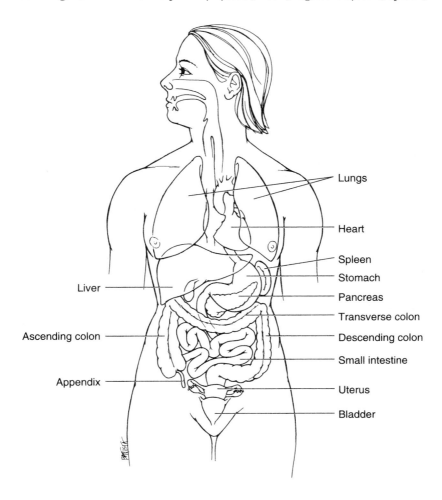

Human torso with visceral organs.

urinary tract, and reproductive organs. It is good to initially explore all of these organs as a group. We can feel the fullness and softness of the visceral organs inside our trunk. On an experiential level, the organs initially present as one big group.

All the viscera have the function of processing our material intake. This includes such activities as mechanical and chemical breakdown, transportation, absorption, extraction, and storage. The internal organs are either hollow, in which case they are composed of visceral muscle, or they are "solid," in which case they are dense with capillary beds to allow for fluid exchange. Their level of activity is controlled in part by the parasympathetic branch of the autonomic nervous system, which regulates internal functioning. This function is balanced with the sympathetic branch, which makes energy available for external functioning. The experience of becoming sleepy after a meal is an example of parasympathetic dominance. If the doorbell suddenly rings, the balance would shift and digestion would be slowed down. Sympathetic dominance would enable us to use our full energetic resources to meet the challenges of the outside world.

As you are sitting, close your eyes and turn your attention inside. Feel your mouth and your throat, and then feel/visualize the organs of the trunk, all the way through the chest, belly, and pelvis. Make a low, humming noise, changing pitch. Use this sound as a searchlight, exploring the feeling of fullness inside your trunk. Take as long as you wish with this. Notice if you have slowed down, or if the quality of your state of mind has shifted at all with this attention.

Psychologically, attention to the internal organs is related to attending to our own personal needs. This is on both a material and a nonmaterial level. We are all familiar with visceral reactions that are emotional rather than purely functional, like "butterflies in the stomach," heartache, or any sort of "gut reaction." Linguistically, we find ample extensions of physical function into the emotional realm. The expressions "finding something palatable" or "bilious with anger" both associate an emotional experience with a particular body part. Cohen (1987) describes the organ system as underlying "feelings, expression, and sense of volume." Most people are able to distinguish a boundary between outer behavior and "how I feel on the inside." The organs are what is "on the inside."

Just as the organs process our physical intake, so do they process our experiences of the world. For example, our small intestines absorb the nutrition we have taken in. Often, difficulty with receiving emotionally is experienced in the small intestines. Oriental medicine has a highly developed approach that correlates the functioning of the visceral organs with emotion.

How much or how little an individual attends to the internal organs varies tremendously. Some people literally feel "hollow and empty inside," which speaks of alienation from their innermost personal reactions. On the other end of the spectrum, some people feel "stuffed" full and unable to process. Culturally we are taught to ignore our organs unless they need medical attention. This is carried to the point that we are ignorant about where they are and what they do. How ironic it is that, in a culture that prides itself on knowledge, most people don't really know where their kidneys are or what they do. We erroneously call the small intestines the stomach, and often the adjectives that we use to describe our sensations are very primitive. "My stomach feels bad" or is "upset" or "hurts." On the other hand, some people intuitively rely on their gut-level reactions, allowing these to inform their view of the world and shape their behavior.

Individual visceral responses to situations are both universal and unique. Many people might respond to seeing an old friend by feeling warmth in the heart area; others might experience an expansion in the abdomen. There are no formulas, but there are commonalities. Fear responses vary individually and situationally; they include tightening of the throat, rigidification of the chest, and knotting of the intestines. Looking closely at each particular situation, it is often possible to find a personal logic that connects past associations with particular organ functioning. For example, the intestines, as mentioned before, are involved with absorbing nutrients. Expansion of the small intestines may allow them more facile absorption. Seeing a friend who has in the past been nurturing to you might provoke this response.

Habituation of these gestural responses in the viscera may lead to organ disease. Generally, when an organ response is not felt, responded to, or allowed to complete its action, the response persists. For example, having a fearful reaction to someone on a gut level but feeling compelled to outwardly trust them might result in a chronic spasticity or lack of circulation in a particular area. Maintained over time, this gesture might result in disease. The responses of the organ system provide an important link between emotional and physical health. The following case will illustrate that link.

Delia was completing a divorce and simultaneously seeking to find her own personal direction in life. She had previously defined herself by her family's needs, which she had met by being "happy, a good mother, and hard-working." Now, at the beginning of a new phase of her life, she encountered sadness and anger. As these feelings arose, she quickly repressed them. If she began to cry she remembered her mother's disapproval and warnings that "her face would freeze that way" if she cried. Instead, she clenched her jaw, tightened her throat, and constricted her lung tissue. Delia suffered from chronic bronchitis, and she im-

mediately felt the connection between that condition and this gesture of not crying. In fact, she both cried and coughed as she realized the connection. This realization became an important gate to her inner feelings. Delia slowly developed a greater ability to perceive and allow her emotional responses, which themselves became a springboard for discovering meaningful direction in her new life.

Regaining awareness of an ignored organ-system response may come slowly. Through our childhood we may have systematically cultivated an ability to ignore these responses and plunge ahead with externally rewarded behavior. Time and conviction are required to cultivate sensitivity to our innermost self. In this case, the insight into the connection between a visceral gesture and a chronic ailment was dramatic enough to convince Delia to pursue a relationship with that part of herself. This involves the body-mind integration principles of respect and, eventually, full participation. With full participation of her lungs, this woman might discover a greater inspiration for the next phase of her life.

In general, sequencing is a very important principle in working with organs as well. Because the organs are deep inside us, they need the support of other tissues to communicate with the world. If my stomach experiences hunger, my brain needs to recognize this and my musculoskeletal system needs to move toward a food source. This requires sequencing within and between the body systems. Likewise, if I experience expansion around my heart when I see you but I do not allow this to sequence, I will not express this warmth in my face or in the gesture of my arms or in moving toward you. Sequencing is required for the health of the organism and to create a healthy and honest relationship with the world.

In addition to experiencing the fullness of our visceral organs as a community, we can become better acquainted with the rich multiplicity of personalities in each organ. There are also experiences, qualities, and responses intrinsic to each organ. In the following pages, we'll explore these individual viscera.

BREATH AND THE ORGANS OF RESPIRATION

The ongoing rhythm of inhaling and exhaling underlies every moment of our lives. Breath is important to every aspect of our physical being. Every sensation and physiological activity has a motivation to breathe in a particular way—whether a long deep breath, a delayed exhalation, or a quick shallow breath. Each breath is an integrated response to the myriad impulses that move through us in any moment.

There is a simplistic tendency to think that there is a correct way to breathe. In fact, different ways of breathing are appropriate at different moments. For this reason, my primary instruction around breath is to allow it. Let go of your breath and allow it to come and go as your bodymind's activities dictate.

Often we control our breath with our nervous system as a way to manage the impression we are making on others or as a way to control our overall energy level. As a particular type of control becomes habituated, our muscles become the stewards of this habit. If we do not want to feel a part of ourselves, we avoid moving it with our breathing. We also avoid emotional states by avoiding a particular way of breathing. This is illustrated in Delia's story: to avoid her sadness, she constricted her breathing. Habitual patterns around breathing are often unconscious and deeply woven into the fabric of our daily lives.

The breath is a function which is subject to both conscious and unconscious controls. Because of this, it has an interesting role in the dialogue between our conscious and unconscious selves. In order to allow our habitual breathing patterns to shift, we must use a very light touch—not overly directive or manipulative. One way to do this is to open your mouth. The muscles around the mouth and lips are often used to control a breath. If you open your mouth, you disarm this control and often your breathing shifts, allowing physiological processes to dictate the rhythm and quantity of respiration that suits them.

Another way to gently allow the breath to become more suited to your physiological needs is to yield in each of the main areas that are involved in breathing—your head, throat, chest, belly, and pelvic floor. The actual air

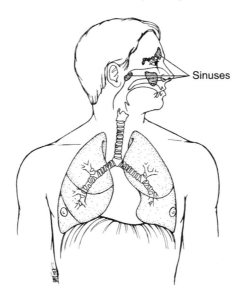

Air passages of head, throat, and chest with diaphragm at base.

passages of our body extend from our nose and mouth into our sinuses, nasal and oral cavities, through our pharynx, larynx, trachea, and down into our lungs. The movement of the breath extends beyond these areas in order to make more room for them to expand with inhalation. As we inhale strongly through our sinuses, our brain is gently and minutely pressed upward. The sutures of our cranium microscopically shift. Likewise, if we allow it, our diaphragm pushes down into the organs below, shifting the position of our pelvis with each breath. As the bones of our trunk shift, they effect changes in our limbs. Thus we have the feeling that our breath can subtly extend all the way into our hands and feet.

 Sitting or standing upright, soften your vision, open your mouth, and breathe strongly into your sinuses. Allow your head to yield as the inhalation fills it.

With your mouth still open, make a throaty sound. Sticking out your tongue, feel your breath move gently through your throat.

Consciously direct your breath into all different parts of your chest. Your lungs extend in points all the way up to your first rib which is under your clavicle (collar bone). See if you can breathe into the uppermost tip

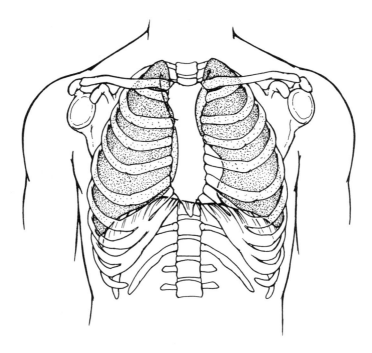

Upper lungs with skeletal landmarks and diaphragm.

of your lungs. Massage around the base of your rib cage from your sternum all the way to your spine. This is where your diaphragm attaches. Breathe in a way that allows the diaphragm to move downward with your inhalation, all the way around.

Squeeze your pelvic floor, and then right before you inhale, allow it to relax. Intend to allow your pelvic organs to rest down, making more room for your inhalation. The feeling is that your breath is filling up your trunk starting from your pelvic floor up.

This is how your whole trunk is involved in respiration. All of the muscles of your trunk can be used to allow your trunk to expand with your inhalation and to rest back into center during exhalation. Thus, a full breath would involve all of these parts, but even a smaller breath could involve your whole trunk in a less extreme way. In this way you can make each part of you available to your breathing process. Nonetheless, it is important to allow your body to breathe in its own way in each moment, only gently offering options.

The lungs, our primary organs of respiration, are not hollow air bags as many people imagine. They are a bloodfilled tissue similar to liver tissue. It is important to experience the fullness of your lung tissue and to allow your lungs to express their particular emotional qualities. We have numerous linguistic connections between lungs and spirit—inspiration, respiration, et cetera. This connection is also acknowledged in oriental medicine which associates the lungs with the polar emotions of inspiration and grief. On a very concrete level, opening up to our lungs and allowing more breath enlivens our spirits.

Our breathing massages all of our visceral organs. The pericardium, the connective tissue which contains the heart, and the pleurae which contain the lungs and their surrounding fluid grow into the tissue of the diaphragm, so that they are attached together. This means that as the diaphragm moves up and down, the pericardium and the pleurae are stretched and squeezed. Think of the image of a small animal moving from a crouch into an extended leap. Taking a deep breathe, imagine these shapes changing in your chest. Underneath the diaphragm, the abdominal organs are nestled unattached. These organs are gently compressed as we inhale.

While the lungs are the primary organ of external respiration (breathing), internal respiration takes place at the level of the cell membrane, as an exchange of gases takes place through the membrane. This is cellular breathing, which is discussed in detail in the next chapter. For now, as you breathe, imagine that your cell membranes are softening and becoming more permeable, bringing oxygen into your tissue wherever it's needed.

Oxygen is a constant source of energy in our lives, free and almost always available. Yet my experience is that most adult Americans are oxygen-deprived. We diminish our oxygen level to limit our creative energy. Open your mouth and breathe! Are you willing to have more energy in your life? What will you do with it?

HEART

The heart is nestled between the lungs as if being embraced on either side. It is an amazing organ that has both neurological and endocrine components. In the sinoaterial node, the heart generates impulses which, combined with external neurological input, regulate the rhythm of cardiac muscular contractions. The heart produces hormones which are involved in blood pressure regulation. As research continues other hormonal functions may be identified.

In our common language, we use the word for heart in many different ways that are both psychologically and spiritually important. For example, we say that we feel profound emotions deeply within our hearts. The most intimate of

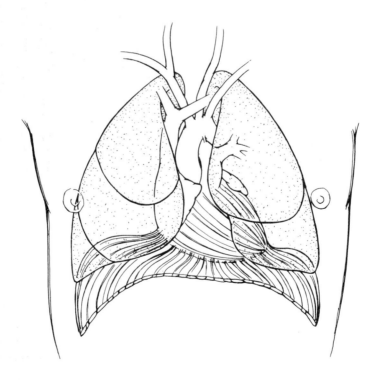

Heart, lungs, and diaphragm in relationship.
Note interdigitation of pericardium with diaphragm.

conversations is a heart-to-heart talk. When we are touched by a spiritual truth, our hearts open. In most Asian languages, the word for *heart* is synonomous with the word for *mind*. This is in contrast with Western languages which equate the brain with the mind. In all cultures, the heart is the seat of powerful emotions. Eastern cultures associate the heart with joy and sadness. In the West, we associate the heart with love, courage, and vigor. What is this potential of the heart that seems to take it beyond the level of our other organs?

One answer lies in its electromagnetic field. Hearts emit the strongest electromagnetic field in the body, 5000 times stronger than that of the brain. Thus, they have the potential to entrain other electromagnetic fields both within ourselves and in others. This may be a powerful way in which states of compassion are transmitted from person to person.

An important psychological lesson can be learned from considering the physiology of the heart. As the heart receives oxygenated blood from the lungs, its arteries receive that blood and distribute it directly to the heart tissue. Thus, the heart that is constantly pumping blood to supply the rest of the body's tissues receives the very nurturing that it gives out directly. This is in contrast to our image of caregivers that acts as martyrs, not fully nurturing themselves before giving to others.

As you can see, our biological/metaphorical heart is a very powerful entity. Researchers at the Institute of HeartMath in Boulder Creek, California are teaching people very simple meditations connecting breathing and positive thoughts to a focus in the heart area. They are getting dramatic physiological results: major increases in DHEA (a popular "anti-aging" hormone), decreases in cortisol (a stress hormone), general improvements in the health of patients with cardiac histories, and general psychological improvements.

Sit quietly for a moment. Let go of your breath. Allow your posture to settle. Feel your heart and feel/imagine that the weight of your head and brain is yielding down and resting into your heart. Open your mouth somewhat and allow your heart to breathe as fully as it wants to. Take a moment to identify a positive feeling such as love or joy. To do this you might think of a particular person or situation that is connected to this feeling. Take a few moments to meditate on that feeling. Have the image that as you breathe, you are circulating that feeling through your heart. As the feeling grows, allow a sense that the feeling is radiating out from your heart.

To go a step further with this, take a moment to identify a difficult situation in your life. When you fix on it, notice if there is any subtle shift in your heart's energy. Then, holding that situation in your mind, go back to breathing love or joy through your heart. Feel/imagine that you are diffusing the difficult situation with your heart's energy. Spend a few minutes this way.

DIGESTIVE SYSTEM

The tube of our digestive tract begins at the mouth. It continues through the throat to the esophagus, which rests behind the heart and lungs and joins the stomach just to the left of the midline of the body. If you place your fingers a bit below the base of your rib cage, in the center of the left side, and press down and in, you will come to an indentation which may be the base of your stomach. Depending on how full your stomach is, it can extend down a couple of inches below the rib cage, or as far down as your pubic bone. The stomach is where we receive our food, and thus has a relationship to our emotional ability to receive as well. In oriental medicine, it is associated with sympathy.

The next portion of the digestive tract is the small intestine. It attaches to the stomach just to the right of midline fairly close to the base of the sternum. The center of our bellies, the small intestine, absorbs the bulk of our

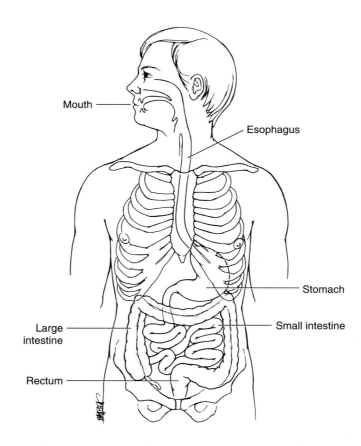

Gastrointestinal tract from the front with skeletal landmarks.

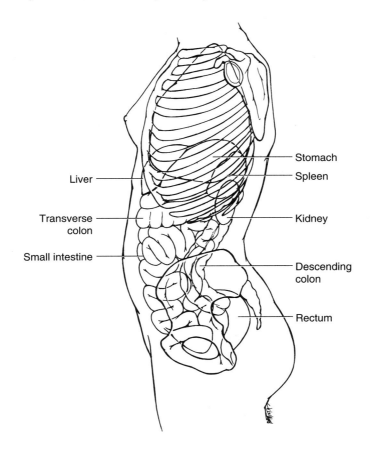

Abdominal organs from the side with skeletal landmarks.

nutrients. Thus, emotionally, the small intestine can be related to the ability to actually absorb, to "take in" what we receive. Often when people say that their stomachs hurt, they are referring to their small intestines. By actually locating the position of your organs and knowing their basic functions, you can better understand the sensations you receive.

The large intestine attaches to the small intestine on the lower right side of our bellies—for most people, a couple of inches below the bony protrusion of the top of the pelvis (the anterior superior iliac spine). From there, the ascending colon goes up the right side of the abdomen. The transverse colon garlands across the front of the abdomen just below the base of the ribs. This is where the bulk of fluids and minerals are absorbed. The descending colon goes down the left side of the body, then loops up and behind the bladder. Finally, the rectum runs down along the sacrum to the anus.

In Oriental medicine, the colon is said to separate the pure from the impure. It is popular in Western culture to equate the colon with control, since quite literally the colon does contain and control our bowels. Understandably, our history with toilet training may be critical to our relationship with our colons. Our ability to control the muscles of our anal sphincter independently does not really develop until about age two. So enforced toilet training before that time may require us to tense most of the muscles in our pelvis. This pattern may persist into adulthood and render our pelvic muscles somewhat unable to release without retraining. Whether this sort of long-term pattern exists or not, fear and control may affect the energetic flow through our large intestine.

Our gastrointestinal (GI) tract is often referred to as a tube within a tube, outside space within the body. It is not until food and liquid pass through the membranes of some portion of the GI tract that they are really part of our bodies. Also it is important to note that there is air in the space within the GI tract. In contrast, inside the body proper, any space is filled with fluid. There is no air space between organs of the body. They generally nestle together.

Outside of the GI tract, the organs that assist in digestion are the liver, the gall bladder, and the pancreas. The liver is the largest of all the abdominal organs, filling the whole area under the right side of the diaphragm. All of the nutrient-rich blood coming from the intestines goes first to the liver which both detoxifies the blood and absorbs many of the nutrients within it. From these nutrients it metabolizes the carbohydrates, producing glucose. The liver absorbs the fats, or lipids, from the blood and from those produces triglycerides, cholesterol, and ketone bodies. The liver also synthesizes proteins as well. Finally, the liver produces bile and secretes it into the gallbladder where it is stored. During digestion, the gall bladder releases bile into the small intestine.

Both the liver and the gall bladder are associated with anger and decision-making in Oriental medicine. Anger is also our Western association with these organs as reflected in the terms "livid" and "bilious." In many hunting and warrior traditions, the liver was seen as the center of power of the dead animal or enemy and thus eaten soon after death.

The pancreas is located below the diaphragm in the center of the body between the stomach and the liver. It has both an exocrine and an endocrine function. As an exocrine gland, it secretes digestive enzymes into the small intestine. In its endocrine function, it regulates blood-sugar levels. The pancreas' location right in the center of the mass of the body has a certain self-existing power. Breathing into that area can both strengthen and center the sense of the whole self.

SPLEEN

A small, quiet organ nestled behind the stomach just under the diaphragm on the left side of the body, the spleen is primarily part of the immune system. It assists in producing lymphocytes, and filters the blood of foreign particles, cellular debris, and old red blood cells. In addition to its immune functions, it serves as a reservoir for blood. When there is the need for extra blood, it squeezes this extra blood out into the general circulation. The spleen generally has very subtle, quiet sensations and does not attract a great deal of attention or express much emotional material. However, in Oriental medicine the spleen is said to be the source of life for the other organs.

URINARY TRACT

The urinary tract consists of the kidneys, the ureters, and the bladder. The kidneys rest in the back of the body outside the peritoneum, the connective tissue container that ensheathes the rest of the abdominal organs. Thus, the kidneys are more exposed to the temperature outside the body. They rest just below the diaphragm on either side of the spine, an area that is often tender to the touch. Find the base of your rib cage on either side of your spinal muscles. This is the general area of the kidneys. The kidneys filter the blood which produces urine which travels down the ureters to the bladder. The bladder rests behind the pubic bone. Find your pubic bone and then move your fingers upward from your pubic bone as you press gently into your body. If you feel a crevice that is probably the top of your bladder. Urine leave the body through the urethra.

Both the kidney and the bladder are associated with the extremes of fear and peaceful flow in Oriental medicine. Some systems of psychoanalytic development identify a urethral stage in between the anal and genital stages. This stage is associated with dependence. A neurotic disturbance at this stage may result in dependent, whiny behavior.

REPRODUCTIVE SYSTEM

While the reproductive system is central to the endocrine system, it is also experienced as part of the general body of organs filling our trunks. This is more true for females than males. For females, the ovaries, uterus, and vagina are part of the contents of the pelvic cavity. The ovaries and the uterus are located behind the intestines. The vagina rests in between the bladder and the rectum. It is important to note that in the male, the bladder and the rectum rest together. There is no gap between them. The male pelvis is still full.

Functionally, our reproductive system represents our ability to procreate. Thus, on an emotional level, this part of us may be generally associated with creativity. The qualities of excitement and ripeness associated with creativity are textures created by the hormonal function of our reproductive system. On the other hand, a simple quality of relaxation in our genitals can allow us to include them more in our everyday life. Feeling the weight and existence of our genitals can be a way to access this. Often developmentally, there may be a self-consciousness or confusion about gender. The ability to acknowledge ourselves as mature women or men embodying a variety of both masculine and feminine qualities is a level of maturity that rests on accepting and allowing our reproductive system to both function and creatively flourish.

Amanda bounced about with so much youth and vitality that her tiny form seemed almost weightless. Yet she revealed a deep sadness underneath that outer persona. Though still young, she despaired of ever having children. After a recent break-up with her "true love," she felt she had lost her chance. She began having nightmares involving him from which she'd wake up in a sweat. This led her to seek counseling. Speaking of how frightened she was in the dream, she sobbed deeply. Her language began to shift subtly, as if she was saying that she was also frightened of him in reality. This contrasted greatly with the extremely positive light in which she had cast their relationship. She began to remember that he had violently threatened her at times. She realized that she had never told anyone and had ascribed that behavior to his wonderfully passionate nature which she so appreciated. Slowly she began to admit to herself that those times were quite traumatic for her. She had frozen a place deep inside her core. She covered up this deep fear by becoming even more bouncy and lively on the outside.

Over a number of sessions, she discovered that this frozen fear had affected her sexuality. She felt numb in her pelvis. As she began to breathe life into it and give it permission to move, she encountered an even older trauma. She remembered her first experience of sexual intercourse. As a teenager, she had fallen in love with her older cousin. With her consent, they ended up naked in a hay loft. She realized that while she had participated willingly, she had been dissociated from her body and had lost her virginity in a semi-conscious state. Reenacting the situation, she felt the numbness in her body. She relived the scenario, changing it by giving her body more permission to respond from its sensations. She imagined pushing him away from her and saying, "This isn't right. This doesn't feel good." She drew the warm hay up around her nakedness and sent him climbing down the ladder. She imagined laying in the hay and holding her belly, as she cried softly. She realized it was this part of herself that she had despaired of ever birthing.

Often our creativity, sexuality, and fertility are all intertangled. A clear relationship with one's pelvis and reproductive organs can reveal these entanglements. Breathing into one's pelvis and inviting its sensation and aliveness in all different situations can give one a base from which to express creativity in all its forms.

Skin

Our skin is our most obvious natural boundary. It is what contains all of us. It is the clearest marker between inside and outside. On the other hand, skin contains us with a degree of permeability, allowing for a certain amount of fluid and chemical exchange with the world.

Early embryos, before we folding into a tube shape, are pancake-shaped, with three layers of tissue. One layer, the ectoderm, is the tissue out of which both the nervous system and the skin develops. So our skin is very closely related to our nervous system. It has a major sensory function; it gathers information about the tactile world and the electrical field around us. Skin is very sensitive. A good deal of our sensitivity is connected to feeling alive and awake in our skin.

 In a comfortable position, allow yourself to breathe however you would like to, and begin to sense your skin. Notice the areas of skin that you can clearly sense and the areas that are less clear. Begin to touch your skin, changing the pressure and quality of your touch as it suits the different parts of you. Touch every bit of your skin from your scalp to your soles. Touch as much as you want to.

When you feel complete, notice how touching your skin has affected the circulation of energy through your body. Notice how it has affected the feeling of flow in your body and your sense of well-being. The skin is central to our experiences of receiving nurturing, to our sense of pleasure, and to our sense of having a boundary. In working with people who are experiencing a lack of boundary, I often encourage them to touch their skin. Waking up the skin can strengthen the experience of having a natural boundary, not one that you have to create artificially but a naturally existing one that is always present.

Touch and pressure on the skin also have an important physiological function. Most mammals lick their infants after birth, an action that triggers important physiological events. Touch can help ground intensity. The pressure seems to help metabolize hormonal activity. I have had many people tell me how much they craved touch in adolescence. Touch helps adolescents ground all the hormonal changes they are experiencing. Family and friends can support burgeoning adolescent sexuality to unfold in a healthy way by giving their adolescent lots of satisfying, nonsexual touch. The following situation involving skin brings together relationship, boundary, nurturing, and sexuality issues.

 In exploring his confusion about establishing healthy relationships with women, Derrick was working to learn to differentiate his own experiences from those of women he was contacting intimately. I suggested he try touching his skin and

talking to himself about this boundary: "Everything I feel inside here is me. Everything I see and hear and touch outside my skin is other." He began with a sense of almost macho indifference. When I pointed this out, he acknowledged this feeling. I encouraged him to really feel and express this attitude. He began saying, "Yeah, yeah, yeah. This touchy-feely stuff is dumb. This is for girls." When he was really embodying this attitude, I asked him to feel underneath this. What was motivating this attitude? What feelings were underneath it? A rush of panic flared up. Derrick was standing and he crouched over, becoming very still. He felt young and imagined being attacked by his mother and his grandmother and his aunts. Raised in a very matriarchal family, he had known that he felt unaccepted as a male. Now he got a very distinct feeling—the feeling was one of deep fear. Feeling pleasure, feeling his skin was dangerous. He felt protective of his genitals. Above all, he felt the fear of touching his skin.

In working with this experience over time, Derrick was able to learn to breathe through this fear, feel his skin, and open up to pleasure. He understood why his boundaries with women got confused when he shut down his own sense of himself via his skin and his sense of pleasure.

Skin is a very "touchy" subject because it brings up a wealth of loaded issues: boundaries, sexuality, contact, and nurturing. Touch between people can be quite confusing. This is especially true since many of the issues developed preverbally. Self-touch is more nurturing than our culture acknowledges, and can be used very effectively to explore psychological issues.

Fat

Fat has a bad name in our culture. We do not like it and, perhaps as a result of not liking it, we are plagued by it. We forget its positive qualities of storing energy and insulating. Healthy fat is a fluid-filled tissue. Our attention and attitudes affect our circulation patterns a great deal. Perhaps in disliking fat we limit circulation into fatty areas. The irony is that in slowing down circulation, metabolism slows down as well, which would cause us to be more likely to retain fat. In less affluent cultures, fat is the wealth that carries one through a famine. Fat is beautiful and healthy.

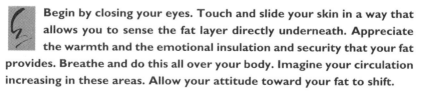 **Begin by closing your eyes. Touch and slide your skin in a way that allows you to sense the fat layer directly underneath. Appreciate the warmth and the emotional insulation and security that your fat provides. Breathe and do this all over your body. Imagine your circulation increasing in these areas. Allow your attitude toward your fat to shift.**

Fat can be complicated by issues of nurturing, both inadequate and excessive. In our culture, food is much more readily available as a source of nurturing than in other cultures. Perhaps it is too available—we all have our mammalian instincts of eating until all the food is gone. This is challenging to contend with when there is an unlimited supply. On the other hand, other forms of nurturing, such as extended family, community, ritual, spirituality, and nature, are less available in this culture. Fat may bring up many issues of nurturing and richness. The following scenario involved these issues.

As an infant, Antonia had nearly starved due to her mother's lack of milk. She had a great deal of panic around any feelings of hunger and, as a result, ate very frequently. She was mildly overweight and newly divorced. Antonia had intense feelings of hatred toward her fat and believed that men were uninterested in her because she was slightly overweight. In an individual therapy session she engaged in an internal dialogue about fat. This dialogue was between the part of herself that was afraid of starvation and the part of herself that was afraid of being without a man. During the dialogue I encouraged her to continue breathing and feeling her fat. As she did this she was able to feel the dilemma that this tissue held. Feeling this dilemma engendered a greater kindness toward herself and more ability to dialogue with herself around these issues. This was especially important in times of loneliness, times when she often reached for food. At these times she would revisit the dialogue and give herself nurturing by breathing and feeling her fat.

Culturally, we are unconscious of how comforting fat is. However, when people visualize an imaginary mother, most of the time they describe her as quite full-bodied. Rarely do people fantasize about being held and comforted by a bony mother figure. By consciously feeling and appreciating our fat, we are more able to balance our conscious and unconscious desires relating to it.

Muscles

The muscles are the only tissue in the body able to change length internally. Other tissues can be stretched or compressed, but muscle tissue actually shortens and lengthens through the sliding of internal filaments. This requires tremendous metabolization of energy as well as a great deal of fluid circulation. The muscles are directed by the peripheral motor nerves and become habituated quickly. Therefore, if the nervous system is often telling a muscle to shorten, it may habituate to a chronically shortened length. The muscles move the bones and cover the skeletal system in a multilayered, multidirectional fashion that is continuous and spiral-like.

Close your eyes. Begin to tense and release your muscles. Notice the continuity from one muscle group to the next, tensing and releasing the muscles all over your body. The movement is like

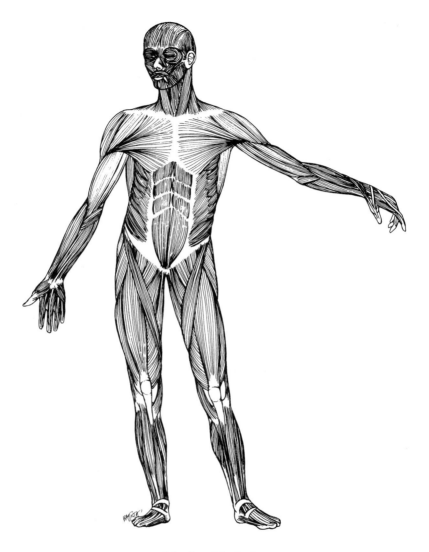

Muscles of the body.

stretching in the morning to wake up or like the movement of a cat. Feel your muscles continuously all over your body. Allow them to move and breathe and sound in their own way, however they want to. Allow the muscles to find their own speed, rhythm, and intensity.

When we identify with the muscles, we identify with our ability to act on the world, to implement change. This might have a quality of perpetual motion, or boundedness, or flaccidity, whatever state the muscles are in. Chronically shortened muscles might bring a sense of being stuck or resistant. Flaccid muscles might have a quality of helplessness. Perpetually moving muscles might relate to a sense of self that is very identified with doing. Cohen (1987) describes the muscles as providing vitality, power, and the dynamics of resistance. On the other hand, a lack of identification with the muscles might relate to feeling ineffectual, prohibited to act, or powerless.

> *The muscles were central to an important session with Jonathan, a 4-year-old boy with cerebral palsy. When he lay on his belly, it was usual for any adults with him to position his hands and forearms in a positive supporting fashion. As I began to do this, he resisted by pulling his elbow back and drawing his shoulder up to his ear. Jonathan also made a sound of frustration and displeasure. I maintained a firm contact with his arm and alternated between lightly resisting his movement and exaggerating it. This created a rhythmical pattern of muscular engagement between us. He continued making his sounds and I countered with sounds of my own. The atmosphere became very charged, not with struggle between us but with an intensity, a fascination, and a sense of respect. His mother was present. We did not speak, but our attention was anchored to the muscular dance that was occurring. The action of drawing the shoulder and elbow alternately in toward the body and then out toward the floor changed in rhythm and range as we continued. The intensity grew until the action was both largest and most violent. At this point, on the outward cycle Jonathan retracted his arm as far as possible and then pushed his hand into the floor. Then he lay his head down on the floor and rested palm open. We all stayed silent as the atmosphere reverberated with the energy of this dance. Finally, he turned toward his mother. She picked him up and held him as we began to talk. This was the first time he performed the action of pushing with his hand into the ground. It was usual for his hands to be in fists, but they pushed flat and open into the ground after this interaction. I remarked to the mother that it had felt like a birth. She was surprised as she had been thinking of his birth the whole time. His birth had been extremely fast and with very strong contractions; there was a possibility that there had been some cranial trauma which had contributed to his susceptibility to the brain infection that had resulted in his cerebral palsy. After this session, Jonathan remained in a state that his mother described as very calm and satisfied.*

In this example, the elements of both ineffectuality (Jonathan could not position his hand to support his body) and resistance (he withdrew his arm when I attempted to position it) were present. When Jonathan retracted his arm, the movement had a very muscular quality, and I responded muscularly. We rode the muscular waves of lengthening and shortening until we arrived at a new capability (push with the hand) and a feeling of satiation. Following this session Jonathan consistently utilized this push to support himself.

This session marked the end of a phase of motivational difficulty in which he was not relating to scholastic, therapeutic, or domestic goals.

Due to the lack of verbal communication, this session might be seen as purely physical in nature, but the emotional impact was inextricably interwoven with the muscular activity. Without a sensitivity to one of these two elements, the body or the mind, this transformation could not have occurred.

In working with muscles it is important to remember their relationship to the nervous system. Muscles are constantly responding to commands from the nervous system, commands that are received both in the form of thoughts and in response to one's relationship to gravity. While the muscles might have their preferences for the kind of movement they like to do, they are constantly being affected by neurological intentions, habits, and gravity.

Bones

The bones are the most solid and enduring tissue of the body. Still they are much more bendable, moist, and alive than we generally conceive them to be. Their substantiality lends support and form to our movement. In general, they have much less sensory capacity than other tissues; similarly, their internal activity is only subtly manifest and slow in completion. The internal activities of bone consist of marrow production and ossification. Bones also dissolve their ossification to provide minerals to the blood. The balance between destruction of old bone tissue and development of new bone tissue is constantly occurring, but at a slower rate than other tissues.

Bones find their health in a balanced relationship to the muscles when they are supported by muscular activity but not obscured by overbound muscle.

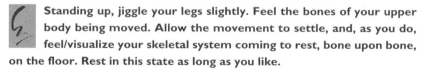 **Standing up, jiggle your legs slightly. Feel the bones of your upper body being moved. Allow the movement to settle, and, as you do, feel/visualize your skeletal system coming to rest, bone upon bone, on the floor. Rest in this state as long as you like.**

Bones can embody stillness and support. Through their joints with other bones, they can also embody movement.

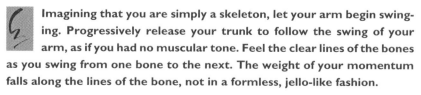 **Imagining that you are simply a skeleton, let your arm begin swinging. Progressively release your trunk to follow the swing of your arm, as if you had no muscular tone. Feel the clear lines of the bones as you swing from one bone to the next. The weight of your momentum falls along the lines of the bone, not in a formless, jello-like fashion.**

Extrapolating these qualities into the psychological realm, we encounter stability, steadiness, and calm, as well as an easygoing quality. Often the skele-

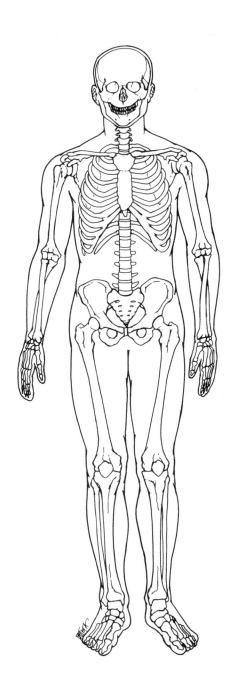

ton is actively involved in a simple "bare bones" sense of support. Conversely, a person may appear to have no bony support when in a scattered, reactive state. Coming back to a sense of the skeleton can ground emotional hysteria. On the other hand, it may be a habitual focus that allows one to ignore emotional needs and responses. Cohen (1987) relates the skeletal system to clarity, effortlessness, and form.

> Tina was constantly struggling financially and time-wise to support herself and her family. This was in conflict with her adventurous nature that was forever leading her into exciting but unsupportive relationships, or enjoyable but depleting escapades. Tina was often in a state of excited desperation. "Support" gradually became an important issue. Support was lacking on a variety of levels—including financial and emotional—and in several directions—that is, from her to her child and to her from her boss, boyfriend(s), and ex-husband. She sought to grapple with her lack of support with the same desperate excitement. In a movement therapy group she rushed about, engaging with one person or activity and then another. Under direction, she intensified this activity. Her speed and her struggle came together in a flurry. There was no evidence of the skeleton in her movement, which was marked by intense muscular and endocrine activity. Finally she collapsed, exhausted, onto the floor. Initially she felt her heart and her breathing, but as these settled, she said she felt like a "bag of bones." Following the suggestion to slowly stack these bones from the bottom up, she took a long time to come to standing. When she did, she just stood. Her expression was very neutral, somewhat blank. Group members had never seen her like this and expressed their amazement. She acknowledged that she couldn't remember feeling "this settled down." She attempted to move about in this state and used awareness to notice when she would "rev up, out of it." In subsequent groups Tina described remembering this state and returning to it during challenges in her life. She used the words, "Just settle down" to help herself find her skeletal support.

This story illustrates awareness of the bones as access to support and neutrality. Conversely, one might feel challenged to emerge from this noncaring skeletal state if it was overly habituated. Emerging would be a matter of discovering impulses from other tissues. The process of this session illustrates that following a state into its logical extreme will allow new qualities to emerge. This is a result of a shift in the balance between the expressive and supportive functions between systems.

Fluids

Fluids comprise up to 75 percent of our total body weight. An ever-changing sea of fluids is constantly circulating through the body, assuming various forms, contents, and functions. As fluid passes through a particular membrane it gains or loses particular qualities. Our body is simply a series of membranes and fluids. As the container changes, so does the shape and pressure it applies on the fluid. Thus, we are constantly circulating a body of fluids that assumes different viscosities, rhythms, contents, and functions. In general, the fluids are involved in circulating contents, regulating temperature, and providing a medium for electrochemical reactions. Each particular fluid carries its particular contents. Constriction and dilation of vessels is one factor controlling the fluid flow. Pressure changes also occur from variation in the pumping action of other tissues, most notably the heart and the muscles. However, through their innate continuity and their pervasiveness, the fluids are a major power in and of themselves.

> **Position yourself comfortably. Close your eyes and let the idea that you are mostly fluid resonate within your body. Feel/imagine that the fluid is only gently contained (rather than rigidly so). Allow your body to soften and melt as the feeling of moistness and fluidity fills more and more of your body. Take as long with this as you like. Allow your body to be rocked by the constant movement of fluid within you. Realize that with all this movement in you, it is an effort to be still. Give in to the flow of the fluids within you. Do this for as long as you like. Notice any shifts in your state of mind.**

Psychologically, the nature of fluid is powerful in a manner that does not rely on control. Transitions are constant and smooth. Outward form may change; internal activity flows steadily. The blood carries nutrients and oxygen through the whole body, eventually supplying them where they are needed. Similarly, fluid goals can be kept in mind almost unconsciously and eventually manifest, seemingly effortlessly. They are not mapped out, scheduled, and forced into existence. Fluid relationships may have a great deal of warmth and connectedness, or they may go beyond this into merging and chaos. Lack of connection to the fluids may result in rigidity or struggle. The phrase, "My blood ran cold," is descriptive of a state in which internal flow is dammed. This literally reflects a sudden constriction of vessels that severely restricts or causes turbulence in the circulation. In order to restrict an impulse toward an action, the first level might be muscular inhibition. However, the restriction of a very strong "hot-blooded" impulse often requires the restriction of one's fluid flow. This occurs at great cost to the individual's sense of inner well-being. Issues of freedom, restriction, and boundaries are often connected to one's style of relating to the fluids. Goals that are approached with fluid support may have a quality of eventual inevitability, as if to say, "We'll get there. Not sure how, but we're bound to get there."

At the start of this ongoing therapy group, Monica had a strong presence and well-developed sense of individuality. However, as the group progressed she began to take a peripheral role and avoid interaction. When issues that angered her arose her response was paralysis and withdrawal. Making contact from this state was very difficult for her, and she remained stuck in it repeatedly. Finally she exposed her dilemma to the group. Monica became angry, but because she could understand the points of view that angered her, she felt she should "rise above" her anger. From this state, being called upon to interact was like being "sucked dry" [her words]. She felt paralyzed and unable to respond. She related this to her childhood interactions with her older siblings and their friends. If they were rough and abusive with her, she needed to "be tough" and not expose her pain or anger; otherwise, she would be rejected by the group. In order to do this, Monica literally stopped her fluids. This state could be observed by a self-inhibition that occurred on a level deeper and more pervasive than the muscles.

The group advised Monica to get her anger out in the open, something she was literally unable to do. This was ironic, as she was generally a very assertive person. Her dilemma was that once she felt directly and personally angered, she would restrict her flow to the point of being frozen. With the help of the group, she recognized her frozen state. Recognition of this frozen state brought her relief. Monica finally experienced it as separate from her cognitive justifications against being angry. She had to first practice expressing anger alone. She found herself "dissolving into tears," sobbing heavily through several weepy days as she began to thaw. Slowly she was able to begin to express direct anger within the group. This broke up the strong inhibition that restricted her circulation when she was angry. After this, Monica could begin to practice new behavior without the physical response of constricting her blood flow.

Fluidity is a powerful force that is largely unconscious in our culture. We operate by a fairly strict time table and spend much time in concrete, wood, and metal rectangular containers we call buildings and cars. Opening up to fluidity can mean opening Pandora's box of the unconscious. Integrating fluidity into our lives requires giving more consideration to open time, transitions, and emotional expression.

As our sea of fluids passes through the various membranes in our bodies it changes name and contents. Entering our body as we drink, we absorb fluid from the large intestine directly into the blood. As blood circulates through the body, it passes through capillary walls and becomes interstitial fluid, the fluid in between the cells. Passing through the cell membrane, our fluids become cellular fluid. Some of the interstitial fluid enters lymph vessels and travels back toward the heart as lymph. Interstitial fluid in the brain passes through a filtering tissue and becomes the cerebrospinal fluid which cushions,

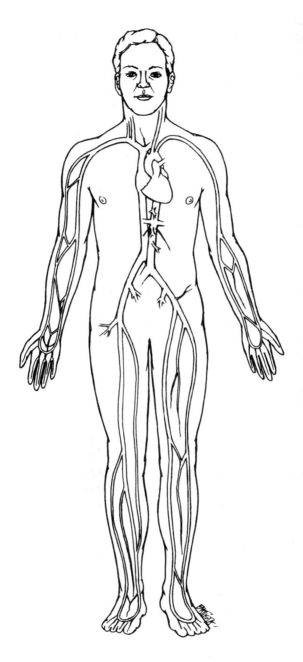

Main vessels of cardiovascular system.

bathes, and nourishes nervous tissue. These are the major fluids in our body. They each have unique qualities, identities, and roles within each of us.

Blood is our thickest fluid, primarily due to red blood cells which make up 44% of its contents. White blood cells account for 1% and the rest is plasma. Like all of our basic body fluids, this plasma is primarily water with small percentages of proteins, acids, and salts. All of our body fluids have a base composition which is very much like sea water. Thus, we are essentially pockets of ocean which have been encapsulated into an organism which can function on land. Biologists Dianna and Mark McMenamin have created a theory of the evolution of terrestrial life which they refer to as *hypersea*. From this point of view, we land creatures have joined together in a network of shared body fluids so that we can exist terrestrially.

We experience blood in two very different ways. As our blood leaves our heart, it has a strong pulse and is moving quickly. This arterial blood has a strong, passionate drive. After you have done some aerobic exercise, notice the feeling that an intense arterial blood flow creates. In contrast, venous blood flow is much smoother. It has a more wave-like sustained rhythm.

Once the blood passes through the capillary walls, it becomes interstitial fluid. At any given moment about 25% of our total bodily fluids are in the tissues as interstitial fluid. Interstitial fluid is circulating in freely between the

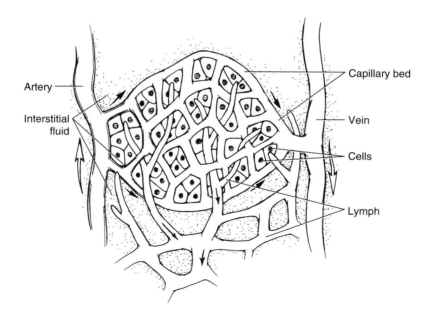

Capillary bed, interstitial fluid, cells, and lymph vessels.

cells. It has an active quality, though it is neither discretely contained nor directional in its movement.

Approximately two-thirds of our total body fluid is in the cells themselves. This fluid is host to the busy metabolic activities occurring within the cell's organelles. Nevertheless, there is a quality to this fluid of having arrived. Alive, pulsating with life, but no where to go, nothing to do.

In contrast, lymph fluid is very directional. It is always headed back toward the heart and it is filled with lymphocytes which have perhaps the most focused sense of directionality of any cell in the body. Lymphocytes head directly to any foreign cells, infection, or injury sites. They are constantly scan-

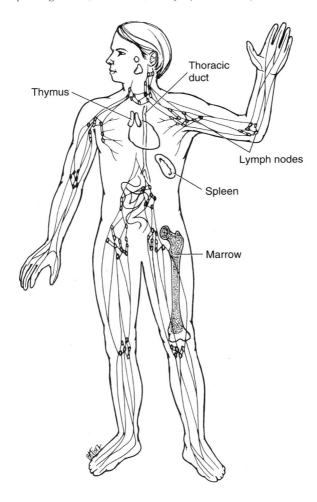

Lymphatic system.

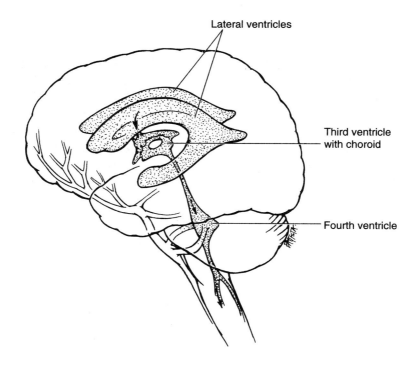

Cerebrospinal fluid circulation through brain ventricles,
and in and around spinal cord.

ning their environment for either immediate danger or signals alerting them
to danger elsewhere. The lymph is often the most viscous fluid in the body
carrying fat and proteins from the intestines whose molecules are too large to
fit in the veins, as well as any refuse from the conquest of the lymphocytes.
Bonnie Cohen likens the focus of the lymph to that of martial arts in which
we are focused on our defense in a fluid, non-rigid state.

The cerebrospinal fluid is a clear watery fluid which filters through masses
of specialized capillaries, the choroid plexuses, into the third ventricle of the
brain. The ventricles are like underground lakes within the brain. Clear, still
bodies of fluid circulate around the brain and spinal cord. Tiny amounts move
out through the spinal nerves and may play a role in providing nutrient ions
to the nerves themselves. The cerebrospinal fluid has a peaceful, meditative
quality existing within our active brain and down the very center of our
spines.

Each fluid has its unique qualities of rhythm, shape, density, and flow. As
you become more and more familiar with an overall sense of fluid flow through
your body, you may begin to notice the signatures of each particular fluid.

The Endocrine System

The endocrine system consists of a series of small glandular bodies that lie, either singularly or in pairs, along the central channel of the trunk, all the way from the top of the head to the base of the spine. They are ductless glands that secrete hormones directly into the blood. The endocrine system controls growth, metabolism, and sexual activity, among other things. More generally, their combined effect could be said to govern overall energy level. Individually, a particular gland or pair of glands may be overactive or underactive. Such an imbalance affects the whole system, which will compensate inter-

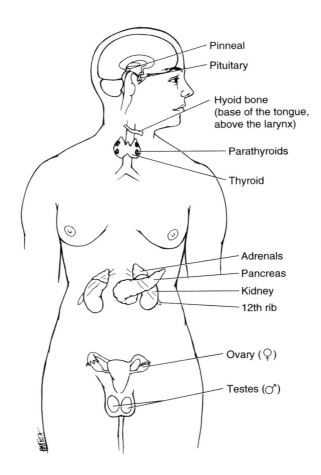

Endocrine system located in head and trunk
with both ribs and kidneys added for aid in location.

nally. Cycles of excitement and fatigue relate to the endocrine system, as do cycles of mania and depression.

Starting at the top of the head, the first endocrine gland we encounter is the pineal gland. The pineal gland, like much of the endocrine system, remains somewhat enshrouded in mystery. At this point, the pineal gland's primary function is in the production of melatonin. Melatonin secretion is inhibited by light and therefore occurs primarily at night. It may play a role in Seasonal Affective Disorder, in which depression occurs in the dark winter months. Melatonin probably plays a role in inhibiting the functioning of the pituitary gland and the gonads (the ovaries and testes). As its functioning is highest from the ages of one to five, and lowest from puberty through adulthood, it may play a role in the onset of puberty.

The next gland in the chain from top to bottom is the pituitary gland. Commonly known as the master gland, the pituitary works in conjunction with the hypothalamus to produce many important hormones including growth hormone; thyroid-stimulating hormone; adrenocorticotropic hormone, which stimulates the adrenal glands; follicle-stimulating hormone and luteinizing hormone, which stimulates the gonads; prolactin, which is involved in lactation; antidiuretic hormone; and oxytocin, which stimulates uterine contractions. Again, these are only the most noticeable hormones secreted and the functions listed here are only the most obvious. Many subtleties of endocrine function are yet to be discovered.

The thyroid gland is located just below the larynx directly in front of the tracheal cartilages and just under the skin. Thus it is very accessible to the touch. Locate your larynx by lifting your chin and pressing on either side of your throat. In this way you will find at the top, the hyoid bone, a horse-shoe–shaped bone which is at the base of the tongue. Just below this you will feel a gap and then below that the larynx and extending from that the trachea. The thyroid affects our overall growth and development as well as the basal metabolic rate of our cells.

The parathyroid glands are four small bodies embedded in the back side of the thyroid gland. The parathyroids are involved in the regulation of calcium balance. They secrete a hormone which promotes a rise in blood calcium levels.

The adrenals are the endocrine glands with which we are perhaps most familiar. They rest on top of the kidneys and are instrumental in the flight-or-fight response as well as any stressful or challenging situation in which we must achieve maximal physical performance. The irony is that in the over-stimulation of modern lifestyle, many people's adrenals are active much of the time. This can result in an ongoing exhaustion and imbalance in the entire endocrine system. In addition to the stress response, the adrenals also work to balance the sodium-potassium ratio in the body, regulate the metabolism of glucose, and produce supplemental sex steroids.

The bulk of the pancreas is devoted to its digestive functions, but throughout it are located small islets of endocrine cells which regulate blood-sugar levels.

The final endocrine glands are the gonads: the ovaries in females and the testes in males. In the fetus, the gonads of both males and females are located in the center of the pelvis, where the ovaries remain. However, the testes migrate through the inguinal canal and into the scrotum. This generally occurs in utero or early infancy. The hormones secreted by the gonads are related both to the reproductive function and to sexual characteristics related to gender. In preparing for sex-change operations, transsexuals are given hormones of the opposite gender. They report major psychological changes often relating to aggression and nurturing. In recognizing the continuum that exists between genders, the balance of various hormone levels is an important factor.

Beyond these specific endocrine glands, there are many other parts of the body which produce hormones, most notably the immune system, the brain, the heart, and the digestive tract. Overall hormonal balance can be said to create a specific texture or tone to our energetic state.

An interesting aspect of the endocrine system is the fact that these small glands that run through the central core of the trunk correspond with the placement of the chakras, or energy centers, identified in yoga and other spiritual disciplines. A Sanskrit word, *chakra* can be translated as *wheel*, designating here a wheel of energy. Different systems have various names to delineate the chakras. Systems derived from Hinduism or Buddhism generally use this term. However, the Judaic Tree of Life and the Native American totem pole have similar centers. Each system has somewhat divergent ideas about the significance of each center; however, direct experience can also provide insight.

The pineal gland can be associated with the crown chakra, which is seen by some as our fundamental connection with the spiritual world. For some systems, this is the site where the soul enters the body. The pituitary gland can be associated with the *third eye* (located between the eyebrows), which is often seen as the source of spiritual power, sight, and intellect. The thyroid gland and the parathyroids are connected to the throat chakra often associated with communication. The thymus and endocrine aspects of the heart are associated with the heart center, which is variously connected with compassion and egolessness. The center around the adrenals and pancreas is associated with a sense of self or ego and worldly power. The gonads are associated with the energy center of sexuality and passion. The root chakra, located at the base of the spine, is associated with groundedness, survival, and basic physicality.There is no endocrine gland at the base of the spine. However, Bonnie

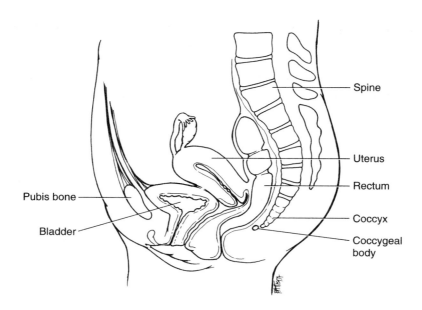

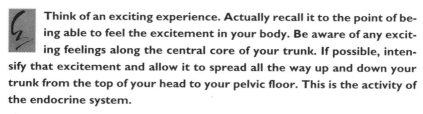

The coccygeal body.

Bainbridge Cohen feels that the coccygeal body, a tiny circular body at the tip of the coccyx, may have an as-yet undiscovered endocrine function.

> **Think of an exciting experience. Actually recall it to the point of being able to feel the excitement in your body. Be aware of any exciting feelings along the central core of your trunk. If possible, intensify that excitement and allow it to spread all the way up and down your trunk from the top of your head to your pelvic floor. This is the activity of the endocrine system.**

The level of excitement with which an individual responds to his internal and external environment involves endocrinal responses. One may be very susceptible to becoming stimulated; prolonged stimulation may result in a balancing swing into fatigue and/or depression. In a depressed endocrine state, it is difficult to be roused by either external or internal events. These states may involve the overall balance of the endocrine system—if one gland is overactive, another might be underactive. The balanced integration of the endocrine system with the rest of our body systems is directly related to our ability to ride cycles of energy and support ourselves within them.

Psychological issues that involve the endocrine system relate to sexuality, gender, spirituality, birth, and power. There are many different qualities, or hormonal recipes, of endocrine states. Endocrine health involves freedom of sequencing from one state to the next, as well as allowing each particular quality of energy to sequence through the entire trunk from the top of the head to the pelvic floor. Often we try to contain our energy. We do not allow it to fully spread through us. This disrupts the dialogue that the endocrine system has with itself and with other systems.

Nita, a middle aged woman with a history of thyroid imbalance within her family, was prematurely gray and had slightly bulging eyes. Nita was extremely bright and had spent most of her adult life bouncing from one intense involvement to another, either relationships or the study of different fields. She sought body-based psychotherapy because she felt she was unable to "ground her energy," and she felt dissatisfied in her relationships. She had a history of relating to mildly depressed men who had problems with substance abuse. Nita was concerned about her mood swings, which alternated between elation and mild depression. She was stable financially and able to maintain a job but did not feel she was "doing anything with her life." In therapy, she first began to experience her mood swings on a physical level as she came to notice the specific sensations involved in her experiences of elation and depression. This led her to be able to detect the shifts before they became full-blown, which consequently allowed her to notice emotional reactions that influenced the shifts. As Nita noticed a shift of mood within her body, she looked for other impulses that occurred along with them. She began to notice muscular impulses to do something in situations where she might habitually have become very still. These impulses generally involved relationship, specifically either establishing boundaries or making intimate contact. As she began to act more on these impulses and express them more muscularly, her mood swings began to self-regulate. She began studying dance and found this to be a grounding outlet for her energy. Slowly, she established more meaningful relationships and pursued a career.

By linking her emotional concerns with her physical state, it was possible for Nita to trace back to a constructive channel for her emotional responses. As she began to make use of this energy, it was no longer tangled up in a self-frustrating cycle. Confusion in the endocrine system often has to do with repressing endocrine-induced impulses or maniacally acting them out. People with a great deal of energy or charisma often have strong endocrine systems, which may initiate a lot of their activity. Children with a lot of endocrine energy are often provoking for adults who have depressed their endocrine energy. These children can become prime targets for parental messages of being "too much." This may mean that the parent cannot tolerate the child's joy, excitement, passion, or power. All of these issues may be related to the endocrine system.

Nervous System

The central nervous system consists of the brain and spinal cord. The central nervous system functions as a major coordination, processing, and control center in the body. From the spinal cord, a paired set of sensory and motor nerves extend from each vertebra. The peripheral nervous system senses stimuli and relays information and motor directions to and from the rest of the body. Via the special senses of taste, touch, smell, hearing, and sight, the nervous system is in direct contact with the external environment. The central nervous system processes this information both consciously and unconsciously so as to determine if an organismic response is required and if so, what response is most beneficial to our organismic goals. The unconscious aspects of this include various cognitive and motor functions. The conscious aspects

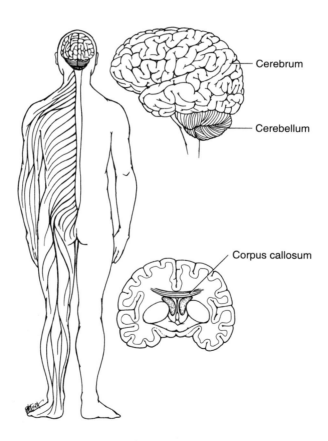

— Cerebrum

— Cerebellum

Corpus callosum

Central and peripheral nervous system.

of this includes our cognitive abilities to think and imagine, both verbally and visually, and move with intention. These are the activities of the cerebral cortex, a fairly recently evolved feature of biological life on the planet.

The nervous system has the ability to monitor, prioritize, and inhibit other functions of the body. It is therefore in a position to take on any role within the polarity of creativity and control. For example, imagine you are nearing a work deadline and every part of you is exhausted and calling for recuperation. As the holder of creative options, the cognitive aspect of the nervous system may respond to this situation in any number of ways. It could crack the whip: "Onward, you knew you only had this much time. Too bad if you're suffering." It could negotiate, "Let's keep going until we're done. Then you can have a vacation." It could attempt to satisfy all the needs, "Here lie down while you work. Have some tea. Stretch your back a bit, and you can keep going." It could take a larger view, "The quality of the work is really deteriorating. It's not going to help anyone to finish on time if the work is poor. Let's make a phone call to postpone, and then sleep on the rest." This is a meager sampling of the various tacks that the cognitive aspect of the nervous system can take in response to its goals and input from the other systems. How the nervous system attends to the conditions and needs of other systems varies individually. The ability to synthesize input and respond creatively varies both individually and culturally.

 To accentuate the activity of the nervous system, notice any sounds occurring around you. Visually scan the environment. Take note of the sensations in your body and your position in your environment. Let your attention shift continuously between these focuses. As if you are scanning your internal and external environment for any important shifts, keep alert. Notice any thoughts that arise and consciously observe the connection between those thoughts and the information you are picking up with your senses. Is there something you should do in response to what you are noticing? . . . Notice if you feel any energetic shift after having done this.

People who rely heavily on the nervous system often neglect the creative intelligence of other impulses in the body. Our culture encourages a lifestyle in which the nervous system may become overworked and lose its clarity. The cognitive function may gradually take on a role of struggling to suppress the rebellious influences of other impulses. "Let's play. Let's rest. Let's get away from this . . ." may be met with, "You're indulgent. You're lazy. You're never going to amount to anything." The most successful relationship of the nervous system to the other systems involves a great deal of flexibility and creativity in incorporating and responding to all the internal input it receives.

In this way, no energy has to be wasted in the process of suppressing and ignoring. Likewise, no alternative resources are neglected.

When the nervous system becomes heavily involved in control through avoidance or suppression, its activity may become dysfunctional, and, in the extreme, delusional.

As an example of this, we will look at the situation of Andrew, a young man working in the mental health field. He entered the field without any personal experience with therapy. This peripheral entry allowed him to slowly assimilate concepts without any personal involvement. He was extremely talkative and seemed unaware that often people were either perplexed or irritated by his style of communication. All of this is indicative of a very dominant nervous system with little input from other systems. After a long period of working within a supervision group that relied heavily on group process, his coworkers began to be direct with him. The pressure he received from them to be genuine and succinct wore away at his verbal defensiveness. Andrew began to remember and communicate about abuse that he endured as a child. Still, his affect was very flat and his discursiveness made it difficult to follow his disclosures. The group employed movement warmups at the beginning of a session, and sometimes did movement within a session. The first time he did a warmup involving the pelvic floor, he nearly fainted. As his memory of sexual abuse surfaced, the group advised him to go into individual therapy. Slowly, as he progressed in that context, his contributions to the group became more meaningful. He began experiencing his bodily responses to what people were saying. Out of this he started attending to and communicating from an emotional level.

The struggle between Andrew's physical/emotional experiences and his verbal/ cognitive defenses became less dense and more apparent. He could actually be aware of the struggle and chose to attend to his present experience. His nervous system was freed from its defensive role of screening his abuse. His logic became more coherent. His ability to take care of himself developed as he grew able to hear and respond to his body's messages, as opposed to repressing and reinterpreting them. His nervous system was integrated in a more balanced way with the rest of the body systems. The movement exercises became less threatening.

Beyond conscious awareness, we can experience the nervous system as a structure within the body. While there are not sensory nerves in the brain, there are more primitive and indirect mechanisms to feel brain tissue. The movement of fluid in and around the brain tissue impacts the surrounding tissue. These tissues sense these pressure changes and we feel those sensations. Also other tissues surrounding the brain mirror the state of brain tissue and we experience the brain indirectly in this way as well. Thus, when we have pushed ourselves cognitively for an overly long period of time we may feel pressure in and around our forehead. Or if we are deeply anxious for a prolonged period of time, we might sense an agitation in the inner core of our brains. In order to feel our brains, we often have to overcome a kind of taboo which places the brain beyond feeling. In addition to that there is always a willingness and openness required to consciously experience any body part for the first time. In addition to these challenges, feeling the brain requires a greater sensitivity since we are feeling it indirectly. Nonetheless, with patience and sensory training, it is accessible to everyone.

> **To feel the frontal lobe of the cerebrum, place one hand on your forehead. Imagine your brain inside and visualize the front of it resting into your hand. Imagine your brain resting down into your hand and, at the same time, rolling slightly down and back to find a neutral resting position. This will feel most dramatic when your are cognitively fatigued.**

To feel the right and left hemispheres of the cerebrum, place your hands on either side of your head. With your hands, move your head in a small figure eight shape, allowing first the left hemisphere and then the right hemispheres to yield into your hands alternately. Feel the balance of yield between the two. Feel the area between the two hemispheres, the corpus callosum (the highway of connections between the two hemispheres). How does this feel in yielding to the figure eight? Imagine/feel both hemispheres yielding down and into center.

To feel the cerebellum, place one hand at the base of the skull. Visualize the cerebellum and rock your skull gently with your hand, encouraging the cerebellum to yield into its own plump, round shape. Often we compress this area.

To feel the brain stem, rock the cerebellum a bit more directly forward to feel the weight of the cerebellum's front side rest into the brain stem.

Feeling the structure of the brain can support the integration the nervous system with the rest of the body. This integration needs to occur on a physical level, as in the exercise above, and on a conceptual level, as well. Often we contrast our bodies with our heads. When we do so, we forget that our brains are part of our bodies. Thinking is a natural function of the human body. The intention of body-mind integration is to balance our marvelous nervous system and utilize it to our greatest potential and health. It is important to appreciate the unique contributions that the nervous system makes to our human existence. Much of our personal uniqueness stems from the particular qualities of our nervous systems. The trick is integrating these qualities in a way that maximizes their resources without overshadowing the possibilities of leadership in the other systems.

The Information System: A Neurocellular System

The physical structures of the nervous system create a series of information pathways. Via these neurological pathways, electrochemical information is passed from one neuron across a synapse to the next. This is one form of neurological processing.

In her book *Molecules of Emotion*, Candace Pert, a neuroscientist, quotes Miles Herkenham, another neuroscientist, as saying, "Less than 2% of neuronal communication actually occurs at the synapse." The other 98% of communication is chemical, from cell to cell via neurotransmitters, peptides, and steroids. These categories of chemicals include many hormones. Francis Schmitt, a neuroscientist at M.I.T., coined the term "information substances" to refer to all these categories. Information substances can be created by any cell in the body in theory, and we know that they are routinely made by many types of cells. Furthermore, they can be received via receptors on the cell membrane by many types of cells.

The information substances bind with receptors on the membranes of cells throughout the body to produce a generalized effect which is both functional and has an emotional tone. For example, oxytocin is a peptide and a hormone and is known to affect uterine contractions, maternal behavior, and long-term monogamy. Candace Pert describes peptides as having a "unifying function coordinating physiology, behavior, and emotions." To visualize a receptor binding with an effector, see a moving torso and head growing out of the cell through its membrane. These are the receptors. A hat floats by. This is the effector. The head and the hat are attracted to each other. Next thing you know, the hat is on the head.

I use the term *information system* to describe this system of communication which includes the nervous system but extends beyond it into a general cellular communication. It is called neurological primarily because of its function of directing shifts and disseminating information.

We experience the information system as an overall experience or state of being with some energetic or emotional tone. This is in contrast to emotional responses that you feel in specific locations in the body. To interact with yourself on this level, 1) recognize the sensations of an overall state of being, 2) recognize the emotional tone associated with these sensations, 3) breathe while you are aware of this. As much as possible breathe in a way that seems to satisfy the state you are in. 4) If you have an overall intention about the state that is respectful and non-manipulative, think this intention while you breathe. For example, if I feel irritated agitation in several general areas throughout my body, I could breathe with it and recognize it. Perhaps it is a familiar state that I know can either gently dissipate or intensify into whole body involvement to the point that my muscles become very tense and my thoughts are angry. Knowing this, as I breathe with the state, I might intend to "Go easy with this and ride it out." Or, for a different example, I might notice an overall anticipatory excitement with which I am familiar from the past. I know that it can intensify to the point that I get bound up in excitement. I might intend to "Ride this intensity gently and allow it to crescendo without becoming overwhelming." I could think that thought as I breathe with awareness of the state. In that case, the state might rework the intention. It might respond with a further thought: "Just trust me. Don't diminish me. I don't have to be overwhelming."

The information system is related to the structural aspects of the nervous system. When neurons, as any individual cell, receive an effector, they communicate this information and a response to it to the rest of the body via nerve pathways. Thus, there is often an important feedback loop between the information system and the linear nervous system. For example, in picking up endorphin activity, our brain will note "Oh, we're in a very euphoric state." This might either intensify the state or begin an attempt to shift it, depending on the overall intentions held by the nervous system.

The information system is closely related to the endocrine system; indeed, in a sense the information system *contains* the endocrine system. However, there are subtle differences between states which are primarily endocrine and states which have functions which are both endocrine and neurological.

Relationship Between Systems

Introducing ourselves to each of the major systems is just the beginning of dialoguing with and encouraging the diverse communications of the body systems. In cultivating a relationship to each system over time, you begin to learn about the events and emotions that have shaped that system's style of existence. Once you become acquainted with each system, you begin to notice the relationships between systems. This is commonly noticed in children when their muscles are extremely active and their endocrine systems become simultaneously stimulated. The result is loud, excited playing. If this energy frightens their caretakers, they may be punished. Over time children may adopt different strategies to avoid punishment, such as avoiding muscular activity or flattening the emotional tone of their muscular activity, causing it to become more mechanical.

It is important to learn about how one transitions between activities in each system. Another common pattern in our culture is that when the nervous system becomes overwhelmed, the endocrine system chimes in with increasing excitement. This leads to the classic frantic stress state that we cultivate in relation to work. How much more effective it is to notice when the nervous system is overwhelmed and invite the fluids to come in and bathe it, providing a balancing contrast.

Another result of our cultural bias against feeling internally is that many people have lost contact with their organs. Our culture is phobic of emotions. Crying is something that other people should not see you do. Only polite, quiet laughter is acceptable. This means that our organs must learn not to fully sequence their energy. We may divert this energy by becoming tight or flaccid in our organs. This might further develop into depressing our endocrine systems or armoring with our muscles. Our creative options for both full sequencing and complete stifling are varied and unique. There is not one particular formula for either expression or repression.

The systems work has much to offer us in the way of integration, valuing diversity, and learning about community and negotiation. Understanding the dynamics of our own internal community can lead to reorganizing in a more creative fashion, allowing us to be more effective and clear. This can clear invisible obstacles for community with those outside of us.

Personal Inquiry and Exploration

As you read this chapter or as you leaf back through it, which systems felt familiar and easily accesible to you? Go through and contemplate each one at a time. As you do this notice your emotional associations with that part of you.

Which systems felt unfamiliar and hard to access? Go through and contemplate each one at a time. As you do this, notice your emotional state as you read or think about each system.

Review each system with the following question: Do you have any history that feels pertinent to your relationship to that system? How do you feel as you remember this history? If any issues around this history were resolved and this system were free to function, how might this system help you in your life right now?

If there are particular systems which you would like to learn more about, get some anatomy and physiology books. In looking at anatomical pictures, try to translate them into living tissue. Always try to visualize the location of any body part in its correct location in your own body. In reading about physiology, ask yourself, "How do I experience this?" The answer may not be readily apparent; you may need to hold this question over a period of time.

CHAPTER 6

Cellular Existence

> Whenever I ask my body what IT wants, all the cells reply, "We are immortal, we want to be immortal," The closer you get to the cell itself, the more it says, "We are immortal."
>
> The Mother, from *The Mind of the Cells*
>
> *The cell is immortal. It is merely the fluid in which it floats that degenerates. Renew this fluid at intervals, give the cells what they require for nutrition and, as far as we know, the pulsation of life may go on forever.*
>
> Alexis Carrel

ALEXIS CARREL WAS A FRENCH SCIENTIST WHO RECEIVED A NOBEL PRIZE IN THE EARLY 1900S FOR KEEPING THE CELLS OF A CHICKEN ALIVE FOR 34 YEARS. THE CELLS EVENTUALLY DIED ONLY BECAUSE OF A CUSTODIAL ERROR MADE BY HIS LAB TECHNICIAN. THE MOTHER (1878–1973) WAS A HIGHLY REALIZED DISCIPLE OF SRI AUROBINDO. HOW IRONIC THAT THE SAME STATEMENT COMES FROM TWO SUCH DISPARATE SOURCES. WHAT IS THE SIGNIFICANCE OF THIS RELATIONSHIP BETWEEN CELLS AND IMMORTALITY?

✺ ✺ ✺

In his book, *Sex and the Origins of Death* (1996), William Clark, a research M.D., points out the fact that unicellular organisms that do not sexually reproduce do not have planned deaths. In the absence of an accidental death (necrosis), they can live indefinitely. The cells of an organism that reproduces sexually, i.e., exchange DNA to create a new genetic identity, are genetically programmed to age and die a planned death (apoptosis). The function of this is to discontinue their genetic strain and make room within the population for the new and potentially improved genes of the next generation. Here again we see a relationship between the cellular level of experience and immortality.

The human fascination with immortality underlies much of our mythology, our cosmological queries, the search for the fountain of youth, and our obsession with longevity. On the one hand, immortality releases us from the biological push to survive, which is the basis of egotistical struggle. On the other hand, mortality lends life a time-limited sweetness and preciousness. How interesting that we mortal organisms are composed of 75 trillion cells which have some connection with immortality. How possible is it to connect to both sides of this polarity by embodying both the human and the cellular levels of consciousness?

Without questioning ourselves, we make simple statements about our cellular state, such as when we say, "I knew it was true in every cell of my body." However, when we consciously think about it we may reject the idea of cellular consciousness. Logically, we may reason that we can think only with our brains; however, biology has disproved this logic. The new science of psychoneuroimmunology has discovered that we "think" with every cell in our bodies. The chemical analogs of thought, such as neuropeptides, can be both synthesized and received by every cell in our bodies. Our cells are highly intelligent entities that can read and respond to a multiplicity of signals, even new signals never before encountered (Kordon, 1993). This is the information system discussed in the previous chapter. Our new understanding of this neurocellular information system and other new developments in the world of *cytology*, the study of the cell, are revamping our view of cellular existence. We are recognizing the importance of the cellular level of existence.

What does it mean to experience oneself on a cellular level? Logic might block this as a possibility: "I am conscious of myself through my brain. I can't experience such minute parts." However, this logic is weak. First of all, there is a difference between self-consciousness, which is consciousness of ourselves, and consciousness itself. Secondly, life has existed on this planet for 3.5 billion years. Life existed only in the form of single cells for almost three billion years before multicellular organisms developed. Organisms with cen-

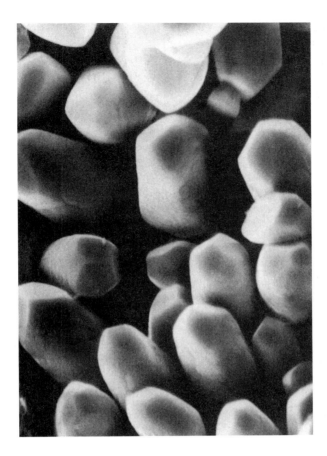

Scanning electron micrograph of human otoconia cells in the inner ear involved in the sensing of movement. Reprinted with permission from Ross MH, Romrell LJ, Kay G. Histology, 3rd ed. Baltimore: Williams & Wilkins, 1994, p. 781.

tral nervous systems have existed for only half a billion years. The human brain as we know it has been around for only ninety thousand years. Ninety thousand is one four-millionths (1/4,000,000) of 3.5 billion. Considering this, is it logical that life could exist mindlessly for so long a time? Can we really equate consciousness with the human brain, an aspect of our physiology that has only been in existence for about ninety thousand years? Do we really believe that all life forms that preceded our highly developed nervous system existed without consciousness?

Dismantling our disbelief in the isolated supremacy of the thinking brain may be the first step toward opening our perception to cellular existence. Imagining the cellular world opens us up to experiencing it.

*In a conversation, cellular biologist Bruce Lipton described to me his en-
try into the cellular realm. After years of marveling at cellular intelligence,
he came to clear intellectual conclusions about the potential for transformation through cellular consciousness. However, it was a purely intellectual belief that he was not really manifesting in his life. One day he was overtaken by
what he at first thought was a hallucination. He found himself in a strange environment, one that took him awhile to recognize. He finally realized that he was
in a fenestrated capillary, an aspect of cellular biology that was a central focus
in his research. He describes that he looked through the openings in the capillary,
". . . and I saw my cells. . .partying!. . . I was furious. Here they were having
a great time and I was suffering. I shook my fist at them and yelled, 'Hey what
are you doing for me?'" At this moment the visual "hallucination" ceased and he
was overcome with physical intensity, writhing on the floor with tremors and
waves of sensations. He says, "This was their answer. They give me sensation so
that I can experience the world." From this experience Lipton felt that it was im-
perative that he take his discoveries more into his life, and so he began lecturing
about cellular consciousness.*

What scientists like Bruce are beginning to understand is that each of our
seventy-five trillion cells is an individually conscious entity. These seventy-
five trillion cells are grouped in many overlapping ways that finally come together as a human organism. In the last chapter we studied the psychology of
our various tissues and fluids. In this chapter, we will go underneath that to
another level of our beings, the cellular level.

The Physical Structure of the Cell

To begin imagining the cellular level of experience, let's look at the composition of a generic cell. There are 256 different cell types in the body, but they
all have the same basic components: a *cell membrane*, which includes gates
and receptors; *cytoplasm*, the fluid within the cell membrane; the *cytoskeleton*; a *nucleus* which contains our genes composed of chromosomes which are
composed of DNA; and numerous *cellular organelles*—miniature organs such
as mitochrondria, endoplasmic reticulum, ribosomes, golgi apparati, lysosomes, and vacuoles.

The **cell membrane** is an amazingly intelligent structure composed of
phospholipids, whose molecules compose themselves in three layers. The
outer layers are lipids that are only soluble in fats, not water, and therefore allow only fat-soluble substances to penetrate the membrane with ease. The inner, phosphate portion is water soluble.

The cellular membrane is not solid. Thus, areas of the membrane can

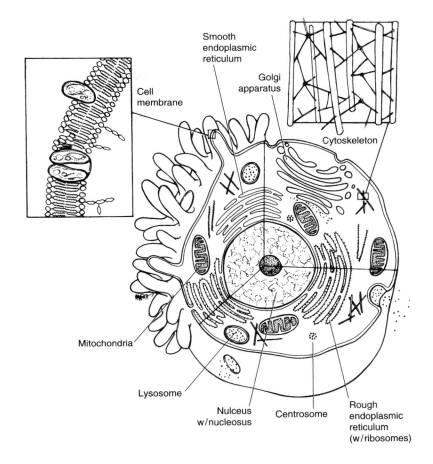

The basic components of every cell.

shift along the surface of the cell. Embedded within the membrane are proteins and carbohydrates. The proteins function as channels for diffusion or active transportation of ions and other water-soluble molecules through the membrane. These protein channels are selective and control what diffuses through the membrane from moment to moment. Proteins which extend into the cell act as enzymes, catalyzing metabolism within the cell. The carbohydrate molecules on the surface of the cell are often receptors for hormones and other information substances. The carbohydrate molecules also act as a link between two cell membranes, attaching cells to one another.

The fluid intelligence of the cell membrane is an example of extremely sophisticated and elegant design within the body. If our organismic boundary modeled itself more consciously after this intelligence, we would grow greatly in our proficiency at negotiating with the external environment. This manifests at four levels: taking in what we need, not taking in what we don't need, sending out what we don't need, and keeping in that with which we are not done.

Within the cell membrane is the **cytoplasm,** the clear fluid of the cell. This is filled with an interconnected lattice of microscopic fibrous tissue called microfilaments, neurofilaments, and microtubules. These are the **cytoskeleton.** The cytoskeleton provides a flexible, but strong structure to maintain the cell's integrity.

The **nucleus** is often described as the control center of the cell and likened to its central nervous system. However, a more apt description might be that it is the library of the cell which contains within its DNA the history of all life and the particular genetic plan of the individual organism. This DNA is activated by the events going on outside the cell, within and around the cell membrane. The cell membrane and its structures are clearly the sense organs and the decision makers of the cell, which send messages to the DNA via RNA regarding what genetic plans should be expressed.

The **mitochrondria** are the "powerhouses" of the cell. Depending on the energy needs of the particular cell, there may be anywhere from under a hundred to several thousand mitochrondria. They oxidize nutrients, producing carbon dioxide, water, and ATP (adenosine triphosphate). ATP is the basic form of available energy within the body and is used by the cell in all important cellular functions. Mitochrondria are self-replicating. Therefore, as we use more energy, they increase in number. The mitochrondria are a good focus for meditative breathing to access seemingly endless energy. Notice the shape of the mitochrondria in the illustration of the cell. Breathe as fully as you wish and imagine the thousands of trillions of mitochrondria in your body, effortlessly expressing themselves by producing energy.

The **endoplasmic reticulum (ER)** both circulates and metabolizes many substances within the cell. **Ribosomes** are attached to some portions of the ER, making it rough ER. Ribosomes function in the synthesis of proteins. The **golgi apparatus** is closely related to the ER. Substances produced in the ER are transported to the golgi apparatus where they are processed to produce **lysosomes.** Lysosomes are dispersed throughout the cytoplasm and provide an intracellular digestive system. They digest all manner of things—damaged cellular structures, food particles, and bacteria.

You should now have some appreciation for the high level of intricate activity that goes on within every cell. This is where change and transformation truly happen within the body.

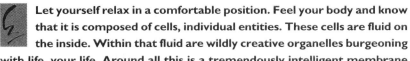

Let yourself relax in a comfortable position. Feel your body and know that it is composed of cells, individual entities. These cells are fluid on the inside. Within that fluid are wildly creative organelles burgeoning with life, your life. Around all this is a tremendously intelligent membrane that is making hundreds of decisions every moment about what comes and goes through it. And then there is fluid surrounding all that. Each cell is constantly communicating with the fluid around it. The cell sends and receives messages—exchanging with the environment, receiving nutrients, sending off the products of its activities that will either be used elsewhere in the organism or will be sent out of the organism to be used by other organisms. All of these exchanges occur through the cell membrane in the form of electrochemical transfers. This is your cell breathing. In these exchanges with the environment, your cells are breathing. All of your cells are fluid with a membrane surrounded by fluid, and they are all breathing, taking in and sending out between these fluids, through the membrane.

Let yourself breathe. Let this image of the cell breathing float around in your awareness. Feel the sensations in your body and follow these sensations to their finest level. Feel more and more deeply into the finest level of sensation and vibration. At the cellular level, the differences in quality between the tissues dissolve. At this level, there is a common experience of subtle vibration. This is cellular respiration. At this level there is a common sensation between your limbs and your trunk, not necessarily uniform, but similar.

Our cells are the basis of all of our physical life. Every physiological event involves cellular activity. Every sensation in our body is the result of these cellular physiological activities. Just as the activities of a country are the accumulated results of the activities of individual citizens, the activities of an organism are the accumulated results of the activities of individual cells. Cytological research is burgeoning right now with an understanding of the body's foundational activity at a cellular level. For example, in the world of nutrition where we previously relied on nutritional supplements that supplied needs on a systemic or a tissue level, we are now discovering supplements that are needed on a cellular or subcellular level. If we can intervene in our functioning on a cellular level, we support functioning on the levels of tissue, system, and organism. This is the basic hierarchy of physiological functioning.

Cellular Breathing

Cellular breathing may be defined as the process of osmosis through the selectively permeable cell membrane and the respiratory and metabolic processes inside the cell. This is the deepest level of communication of information throughout the body. Until a substance or message arrives at a cell, its process is not complete. And in fact, at the cellular level, substances and messages are one and the same. Body and mind are indistinguishable at a molecular level. Within a living organism, the basic unit of both mind and body manifests on the molecular level. Cellular breathing can support any healing or transformational process that is occurring in the body.

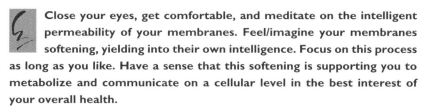 **Close your eyes, get comfortable, and meditate on the intelligent permeability of your membranes. Feel/imagine your membranes softening, yielding into their own intelligence. Focus on this process as long as you like. Have a sense that this softening is supporting you to metabolize and communicate on a cellular level in the best interest of your overall health.**

The Transformational Nature of the Cells

There is a basic relationship between the organism—your whole self—the body systems, and the cell. Each level of being—organism, systems, cells—is an entity within itself, and yet they create a functional and hierarchical community. Each has its own motivation, and yet in integration there is a shared motivation. The role of the cell is at once the most minute and the most fundamental role. When one combines an understanding of the basic role of the cell within the body with an understanding of the range of cellular activity, the transformational possibilities are phenomenal. The range of cellular activity seems at this point in our research to be nearly infinite. There are three general reasons for this.

Cells have a certain level of mutability inherent in their structure. All multicelled organisms are initially one cell. This cell initially multiplies without differentiation. When there are a certain number of cells, the cells begin to migrate and differentiate into different types of cells. The freedom of cells to differentiate into whatever cell type is needed implies a plasticity of structure. The process of cellular differentiation is one of the mysteries biologists are investigating right now. Furthermore, in organisms like the salamander and other simpler forms of animal life, we can observe that cells are able to dedifferentiate and then redifferentiate to regenerate severed body parts. While regeneration of limbs does not occur in humans, the potential for dedifferentiating still exists on a cellular level. **Inherent structural mutability** is the first quality of cells that makes their potential so great.

The second quality that makes cellular potential so phenomenal is that their range of output is broad. For example, although liver cells might be accustomed to their particular activities of storage and breakdown, if called upon they could produce chemicals usually manufactured by the central nervous system or the thyroid gland or virtually any other organ in the body. In other words, every cell has the basic mechanisms in place for producing nearly the entire array of chemicals in the body. This tremendous **plasticity of function** is the second quality of cells that makes their potential so vast.

The third quality of cells that opens up their potential possibilities is their **directed genetic mutability.** Darwin introduced the idea of random genetic mutation and this is still a basic mechanism of evolution. However, new more compelling mechanisms have been discovered. In 1988, biologist John Cairns and his associates at Harvard starved a group of lactose-intolerant bacteria and then gave them a lactose-based food source. An unpredictably large number of these bacteria mutated toward being lactose-tolerant. This and subsequent experiments have posited the possibility of directed mutation. A basic principle in biology is that any characteristic that enhances adaptability will be carried over into further development. Directed mutation certainly appears to be such a trait. The potential ability of directed mutation is the third reason that cellular potential is so great.

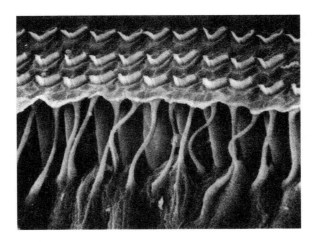

Scanning electron micrograph of phalangeal cells in the inner ear. Reprinted with permission from Ross MH, Romrell LJ, Kay G. Histology, 3rd ed. Baltimore: Williams & Wilkins, 1994, p. 788.

As these three qualities illustrate, our cells hold tremendous possibility for transformation. It is literally true that at the cellular level we can transform— we can change form. My work at the cellular level of experience shows that our cells are tremendously willing to participate in the life and intentions of the rest of the organismic community. They are willing to do the job they are given; they are willing to support the vision of the community. Yet, in this willingness, there can also be a certain docility.

Let's use the metaphor of an employee in a large bureaucratic organization. This employee is very loyal to the company and dutifully performs her job. She uses a certain aspect of her skills to do this particular job. She has many skills that are never utilized within this position, but that is of no concern to her. She identifies with her corporation, its mission, and her job within that: "We are Alpha Corporation and we make thingamabobs and I do THIS step." If her corporation is taken over and undergoes a major identity shift, she is willing and able to transform. "Now we are Beta Corporation and we make doohickeys and I do THAT step. . . . OK, no problem." Now if for some reason the corporation gets interested in this particular employee and asks her to 1) do more than she is doing, 2) change her role, or 3) illuminate some mystery of the corporation's functioning, they might be surprised by the untapped resources in this employee.

This metaphor characterizes the qualities that I repeatedly encounter at a cellular level. Both for myself, in my clients, and with my students, I have experienced these particular qualities: **complete devotion** to the organismic identity, a **single-mindedness** in performing a particular task, and an **ability to transform** both task and identity. Beyond this there is a sort of egoless quality, as if the cells do not get attached to a particular identity. This is consistent with their abilities to mutate and differentiate. This egoless quality is alluded to in the quotation by The Mother at the beginning of this chapter. It is as if our cells will go along with our ego's fixation on survival as long as we are committed to that. However, the cells themselves seem basically egoless in a certain sense.

Cellular Communication

There is another basic way that we experience ourselves cellularly. This is through the totality of the chemical system of peptides and other molecular effectors that communicate on a general level throughout the body. The great discovery of psychoneuroimmunology is that many of the chemical transmitters that we thought of as purely neurological are both generated and received by a variety of cells throughout the body. Francis Schmitt, a neurosci-

entist at MIT, has dubbed these chemical transmitters as "information substances." Candace Pert, currently at Georgetown University and author of
Molecules of Emotion (1997), says that peptides perform a "unifying function—coordinating physiology, behavior, and emotions."

Sometimes we experience an emotion in a particular spot in the body.
Other times, we feel emotion "all over." My guess is when we experience emotion "everywhere," we are experiencing a shift in the informational system of
the peptides.

Tapping into a cellular level can provide a key to transformation. *Breathwork, meditation,* and an *openness to cellular experience* seem to be access points
for tapping into a cellular level. Experiences that radically shift identity, such
as marriage, divorce, sudden job loss, birth, and death (both witnessing and
experiencing death), can spontaneously lead us into a cellular level of experience.

*In facing a divorce, Edward was overwhelmed by the history of failed rela-
tionships in his life and in the lives of his family members. He had worked
to develop a capacity in himself for nurturing relationship, and so his identity was shaken by his impending divorce. Was he, he wondered, doomed by his
family history, incapable of creative and nurturing relationship? I encouraged him
to breathe deeply into himself as he asked this question. As he went deeper and
deeper into himself, Edward went through layers of shakiness to a layer of vibration that was more peaceful. "I feel open to real intimacy," he said. "Good," I
said, "Breathe this into your cells." He breathed even more deeply. Working with
himself on a cellular level, he encountered a great willingness to be intimate. Edward felt creative and nurtured from this place and was able to use it as a support
during the transitions he encountered, both through the divorce and in opening up
to new relationships.*

One of the pitfalls of seeking cellular awareness is the concern, "Is this it?
Am I getting it?" The answer is: it is more important to have an intention
than to have confirmation. The cellular level of experience is subtle, but it is
also an everyday reality. Of course, it may be easier to notice these moments
of cellular experience if you have a lot of experience with your body and your
sensations, but working with the body systems as described in the previous
chapter over a period of time might also facilitate cellular awareness. And the
easiest transmission of recognition of cellular experience occurs within human contact, body to body.

While every cellular experience is different, the hallmarks of the cellular
level of experience seem to be a fine level of sensation that is fairly continuous over large parts of the body, and feelings of permeability, containment,

and constant, subtle energetic activity. As more people consciously experiment with cellular breathing, further understanding will be generated by the unique quality of each person's experience.

> **Pick an issue or area in your life that you would like to transform. Take a very open attitude about it. Try to relax your aggression around transforming. Take the intention of inviting yourself to transform and be open to the response your invitation receives. It may be more important to discover the issues around this intention to transform than to force a change.**
>
> **Once you are clear about your intention, repeat it to yourself as simply and directly as possible. Reduce it to one or two sentences with short words and first-person pronouns, such as, "I want to have access to more energy." Edit out negative statements; for example, change "I don't want to be sick" to "I want to be healthy." Breathe as you repeat this intention to yourself. Feel the shifts that occur in your body as you work with this intention. Be open to whatever arises: images, thoughts, sensations, and movement impulses.**

This sort of intention might lead you into the cellular level of experience or it might lead you into experiences that involve your whole organism or particular systems. Or it might lead you into some combination of these. Whatever occurs, try to accept and appreciate what you receive from this inquiry. Transformation is most accessible when we appreciate the obstacles to it and the mystery that may enshroud it. Bullying cells into transformation is not an option. The very act of such forcing obliterates the openness and the fine level of sensation that is part of a cellular dialogue. Rather, the best catalyst for cellular potential is breath and celebration.

Allow your cells to breathe fully. Cellular breathing can be a catalyst for everything that supports our health. Give them permission to do what they need to do. And celebrate the tremendous mystery and potential that we carry within us, seventy-five trillion times over.

Personal Inquiry and Exploration

Take some time to write about your beliefs regarding 1) the possibilities of cellular consciousness and 2) the importance of cellular consciousness.

Give yourself time to reread the cellular exercises. Try these exercises out and then write about your experiences.

Over a period of time, look for experiences in which you feel sensations that have a cellular quality.

Practice cellular breathing.

Integrating Our Bodies: Healing, Development, and Transformation

All problems are psychological. All solutions are spiritual.

Thomas Hora

. . . AND ALL EXPERIENCES ARE PHYSICAL. HOW CAN WE INTEGRATE THESE LEVELS OF SELF— PHYSICAL, PSYCHOLOGICAL, AND SPIRITUAL— IN A WAY THAT ALLOWS US TO GROW INTO OURSELVES FULLY, TO WALK THE PATH OF BEING HUMAN? THERE ARE MANY INTERRELATED LEV- ELS THAT COALESCE INTO EACH INDIVIDUAL'S PATH. SOME HAVE TO DO WITH HEALING OLD WOUNDS; SOME HAVE TO DO WITH MAKING THE ORDINARY STEPS OF GROWTH; AND SOMETIMES THESE TWO COME TOGETHER IN A WAY THAT FEELS TRANSFORMATIONAL.

❃   ❃   ❃

Healing, development, and transformation are concepts that have many blurred and overlapping definitions. All of them involve movement along a path. Defining these terms more clearly can further their mutual process. The word *heal* has its roots in several early European languages; in each language its meaning is "to make whole." To make whole that which has been divided—the image of skin growing across a wound comes to mind. The word *develop* has moved from its most primitive definition of "to unfold" to the more sophisticated meaning "to become larger, fuller, more mature, or more organized." *Transform* is perhaps the most body-based of all three terms: to change forms, to move from one form into another.

In becoming more organized, we often need to disorganize for a period. This is true for any complex system. In the process of moving toward more wholeness and greater organization, chaos arises. When does a developmental stage of chaos relate to wounding, illness, and fragmentation?

When they overlap, then healing and development are mutual processes. If we focus only on healing the wound, we might miss the larger developmental process that is being facilitated. When we see healing as a part of development, we appreciate the wisdom of chaos and, therefore, the wisdom of the wound or illness. This is the intimate relationship between healing and development.

When development involves the changing of form, we call it transformation. When development involves a systemic shift to another order, we call it evolution. Simultaneously our personal development is embedded in the larger evolutionary process of our species, and our cultural evolution is tied into that as well. Thus all these directions converge within the path of personal development.

Whatever we call it, the development inherent throughout a normal human lifespan challenges a cultural myth. We have been taught that we grow up and become an adult. We expect to be that same adult until we die. Ron Kurtz (1990) illuminates this approach: "First we learn a self and then for the rest of our lives we simply use it. . . . At first we are map makers, then map users." This way of being denies our innate human tendency toward lifelong development. All of the material in this book is pointed toward using our bodies to support ourselves to grow and develop. Putting it all together is the art of working with ourselves. The art of living is inherently about this dance between healing, developing, and transforming. It is a multidimensional and paradoxical dance in which, at times, we go down to come up, and disintegrate to become whole.

 I had the honor of witnessing a very lovely and complex transformational process. Julian had been diagnosed as schizophrenic in his late adolescence, and though he was in his middle thirties, socially he still had a very

adolescent style. He was living at a meditation center, hell-bent on achieving en-lightenment, when he received a diagnosis of visceral cancer so advanced that no treatment was prescribed. He asked that he be allowed to die at the meditation center, and a hospice program was set up for him. He also asked for support in creating a macrobiotic diet, a diet that is known in particular for its successful treatment of cancer. He met with a macrobiotic practitioner and together they created an incredibly pure dietary regimen: rice was soaked in water and sunlight for hours before it was cooked, and then it was hand-ground into cream. Each meal was a careful balance of elements, utterly pure and prepared with great care.

Julian ate this way for several weeks; in that time the cancer progressed to the point that his belly was lumpy and moving and of many different colors. He seemed to enjoy the macrobiotic diet, though he made a few jokes about it. Mean-while he worked with his meditation in preparation for death. His state of mind began to change. At the beginning of this process he was making jokes about kiss-ing girls; toward the end he was noticing subtle worries on the part of his care-takers, and making statements like, "Please don't fight. It is such a waste of en-ergy."

Toward the end of his illness, Julian expressed a great deal of appreciation for his diet, saying, "All my life I wanted to feel pure inside, and now I do." He thanked everyone involved in preparing his food, then said, "Now I would like some straw-berry ice cream." Meanwhile, his belly looked like a war zone. A few days later, a powerful meditation teacher arrived at the center and gave the young man a bless-ing. That night he died. The monks traveling with the teacher said that surely he had become enlightened.

For Julian, transformation did not mean that he was cured of cancer and lived happily ever after. It did mean that he both received and gave new experiences that touched him and those around him to their core.

Transformation involves opening to what is. Often we become confused—we demand what we want and then, when we don't receive it, we collapse in the face of what is. Our natural human ability to imagine, to aspire, and to intend needs to be joined with a healthy grounding in reality. When these two meet, one rides the horse of one's life with a glorious harmony between the horse and rider.

Body Wisdom in Transformation

Approaching life through offering one's aspiration and attending to what arises is a wonderful practice in itself. Our bodies are the ground for this path. Often we fight against our bodies' proclivity to transform. By working within their natural functioning, we garner their intelligence.

ACCEPTING OUR PHYSICAL REALITY

In the bodily world, there is no support for illusory fantasies of transformation. We can feel reality directly and work with it tangibly. I might like the *idea* of remaining calm in a particular situation, but if I feel certain sensations arise in my body in that situation, I cannot deny that I am, in fact, angry. Accepting our physical reality helps us to accept responsibility for our experiences. It is as if one says: "This is *my* life. I can feel it moving through my body. I can feel my own desires. I feel grounded in my body and my reality." This is the grounding that the physical body offers.

Still, there is room for intention. We can intend to go further. We can see the horizon. We can go toward it, working with the experiences we encounter. We can grow the necessary skills and qualities along the way. By feeling our own energetic development, I gain tremendous leverage for pursuing my aspirations. The path of the body is a most tangible and immediate path.

 On a physical level, acceptance can translate into grounding. Grounding means feeling our feet on the ground, allowing the weight to yield through our pelvises and legs and into the ground. Stand up and place both feet evenly beneath you. Gently bounce up and down to release your weight. Allow your breath and voice to release a bit onto the support of your lower body.

On a physical level, intention can mean the willingness to look out. Let your eyes rest back into their sockets which are resting down into the support of the ground. Let yourself look out at the world from eye level. Feel where you are. Look at what is ahead.

OPENING TO OUR DESIRES

"What do I want?" is a very potent developmental question. You may use this question on a very grand scale, as in, "What do I want in my life right now?" or in a very small arena, as in, "What do I want to eat right now?" At any point along this continuum, our bodies can provide us with feedback to this question.

In order to investigate this process, I asked a person with no conscious experience of body-mind integration.

 "Darlene, what do you most want in the world right now?" She snickered, and said half-playfully and half-sarcastically, "A motor home." I said, "OK, think about your motor home—what it looks like, what you would do with it. . . ." Her face softened; her heart area reached forward; there was a very fluid quality in her upper body with a light touch of excitement that had an endocrine tone. I asked her, "How does that feel?" She replied, "Good. . . fun." However,

looking at her body I saw a larger picture. While her upper body had been opening to the idea of the motor home, her lower body had responded by curling back into itself, constricting in her small intestine and becoming flaccid and powerless in her pelvic floor. While her upper body was saying, "Yes," her lower body was saying, "No, I am incapable of that and I won't take it in."

When we are at the edge of our development, there is usually both a "yes" and a "no." That is what makes it an edge. We are not fully there yet. We are flickering back and forth.

Seeing Darlene's lower body response, I queried, "So, can you get one?" First her upper body collapsed out of the reach and down onto her lower body, which was already collapsed. Then she bolted upright with a very strong push in her pelvic floor, and said, "Hell, no." Her pelvis was empowered by her commitment to the negative side of the question. "We'll never have that kind of money." She was putting her powerful push behind the "no," obliterating the half-sequenced reach behind the "yes."

What are the alternatives? Often it is safer or easier to stick with the status quo rather than pursue our own development. Yet the direction for change is clear.

Imagine something that you have wanted in your life for a long time. As you clearly put vision to that longing, imagine yourself in the same position as Darlene was when she was thinking about the R.V. Feel the openness and longing in your heart and the constriction in your belly. Then allow the reach from your heart to fill your whole trunk. Feel it throughout your body. Your eyes and brain could join your heart in reaching. They could look for the possibilities, seek out the direction. Your pelvic floor could join in the reaching. It could sense, "OK, this is where we are now. Where is it we're going?" Your small intestine could open into an absorptive state, moving out of the constriction that cannot take in any nourishment. Imagine a deer sniffing the air, reaching through its whole trunk, curious, open to information. That reach sequences through the whole trunk. Map that onto your own body.

When we mobilize an action and allow it to sequence through the whole body, we access a powerful force that could move us into a new state or stage of development. Each experience involves a particular physical state that includes sensations in particular tissues or systems. As the experience evolves, the physical energy sequences. A developmental action emerges. This moves us through our developmental edge into a new state.

Imagine if Darlene were to say, "Dammit, why not? Why can't we get a motor home? I could start my own agency instead of working for one. I know I could do the job better for less money anyway. We could rent our house." What would be happening in her body? Her eyes would be ablaze. Her brain would be buoyant and reaching with all its inspiration. She'd be breathing fully. All this would sequence down into her pelvic floor, which would respond with a strong affirmative push. "Yes, I'll back you up on this inspiration. I can help get this job done."

Opening to our desires, questions, and aspirations takes courage. Sustaining a reach toward something that is currently out of our reach can leave us feeling excruciatingly vulnerable. We feel safer focusing on what we don't have, habitually dwelling on what is lacking instead of moving toward what we want. In order to move steadily toward what we want, we must continually employ the art of bringing together heaven and earth, bringing together inspiration and practical reality. This brings us to our developmental edge.

WALKING A DEVELOPMENTAL EDGE

As evolving beings, we always have a developmental edge. As a child, I once saw a tidal bore in the Bay of Fundy in Nova Scotia. A tidal bore is a shift from an empty river bed to a full one, based on the tides at the nearby ocean shore. Waiting for it, I had no idea what to expect. We looked across the big, muddy expanse of the waterless bay. In my memory I see a wall of water a yard high come chugging along up the bed; there is a river in its wake.

For me, this is an ideal image of a developmental edge which, as evolving beings, we embody. We chug, we ooze, we flicker between who we were and who we are becoming. Arnold Mindell (1992) describes his view: "An edge is a filter to what you are perceiving. It marks the limits of who you are and what you imagine yourself capable of. . . . Ask yourself if there's something that you want to do but cannot yet do. . . . something in your life that you are almost able to do. . . .in fact you do it occasionally."

We all have developmental edges. Some are active, and others are dormant. We have edges that underlie all of our activity, and edges that are focused on a certain aspect of our lives, such as communication, sexuality, productivity, spirituality. Picture an amoeba: its membrane is a three-dimensional edge. As it oozes out in any direction, its shape changes. If we add both expanding and reorganizing to this amoeba image, we have a primitive visual model of overall human development.

Somehow our culture has fused development and shame, as if the fact that we are developing means we are deficient in some way. This view stunts our development. As soon as we recognize a direction that we could grow in, we feel inadequate that we are not already there. This is contrary to human nature. Human beings are innately oriented toward growth throughout our life-span. As discussed in Chapter 1, we are neotonous—creatures that continue to develop throughout our lifespan. We can take joy in becoming who we will someday be. There is great satisfaction in going with the richness of our ever-changing beings. An old saxophone player was told by his young student, "Man, I'd have to practice my whole life to get to where you are." The teacher responded, "Yes?" Of course, it should take our entire lives to develop the finest parts of ourselves.

We also shame ourselves by comparing our development to that of others or to some linear view of development. There are so many aspects to human development: cognitive, motor, moral, social, and so forth. For these we can discern somewhat sequential stages. However, if we look at the overall life development of the whole person, we do not find linear hierarchies of achievement. It is difficult to compare one person's developmental path to that of another; we are each so unique that one person might grapple in infancy with what another person approaches at death. The sequence and stages of energetic development are unique to each person. Conventionally, we have very limited concepts about human potential, which in turn leads to a limited vision of proper development. That vision usually looks something like this: we are born, we learn to walk by one year, we learn to talk, we go to school, we graduate, we establish a vocation, we get married, we have children, we support ourselves and our children through financial stability. This framework creates a great deal of pressure for those who have different paths. "What's wrong with my kid who isn't talking by age two?" Maybe nothing. Many brilliant thinkers have been too busy observing the world to comment on it. "What's wrong with me that I can't settle down to one career?" Again, maybe nothing. In this age of synthesis, it may take several changes to integrate one's life work. To truly ride the wave of our developmental edge, we must appreciate the unique path we are taking.

We might also feel that, as we mature, we grow out of our previous phase. This is true in some cases, but a great loss in others. As we grow, our repertoire of humanness can expand to include more options. Our body can access all the ages it has ever been—all the qualities of infancy, toddlerhood, childhood, adolescence, young adulthood, adulthood, and eldership. We can feel birth and death. As we navigate through our lives, we have a vast array of options.

And as we ride the waves and eddies of these options, we contemplate our lives and questions arise. We can follow these questions of development down a path of self-condemnation and pathology, or we can follow them to our developmental edge.

Ask yourself, "What am I wanting most in my life right now?" or "What am I wanting in relationship to my work or family or friends?" In response to these questions, feel the flickering quality between the advance and the retreat, the "yes" and the "no." What parts of your body open to your desire? What parts contract? Feel how your body shapes the "yes" and the "no." Feel how much or how little these bodily responses have permission to sequence. Consciously give yourself permission to really feel the sensations that are saying "yes" to your desire. Allow them to move and breathe and spread through your body. Then, consciously give yourself permission to really feel the sensations that are saying "no." These are parts that are afraid or have some genuine concern. Allow them also to move and breathe.

This is how you are embodying your edge. In order for it to be an edge, there is a part of you moving forward and a part holding back. If you were there with your whole heart, there would not be an edge. In these bodily responses we can see powerful internal forces that communicate with the world. Our bodies create the answers to these developmental questions.

ENGAGING IN DIALOGUE

Feeling the "yes" and the "no" responses in our bodies is a potent exercise. By shifting our attention back and forth from one sensation or set of sensations to the other, we begin to create an energetic dialogue. This dialogue may be verbal, an actual conversation between two places in the body, or two states of the whole body. The dialogue may be movement from one posture to another. The dialogue may also be energetic, beginning with a shuttling of attention from one sensation to another until a flow of sensation opens up between them, and they mix and mingle and create a path.

Just as it is a skill to learn to dialogue verbally with another person, it is a skill to learn to dialogue within ourselves. Skill in dialoguing with the outside world needs to be translated into the internal world. The reverse can also be true. Oftentimes people expect internal dialogue to be crude. But, when it is too crude it is ineffective. Through practicing attention to sensation, natural movement, and embodied relationship, we can cultivate our ability to dialogue between the forces moving within us. For Darlene in the example above, her dialogue might be between her longing for fun, her powerful negative limitations, and her disempowered guilt about having fun.

 Again, ask yourself the developmental question: "What do I want in my life (or some aspect of my life) right now?" Hear your answer. Notice how your body is saying "yes" and "no" to this answer.

Spend time with each set of responses. See if they have any words or images to share. Shuttle back and forth between the different sets of responses. Let a conversation emerge, whether verbally, in movement, energetically, or all three. What are you learning about your current situation? What are you learning about the forces within you for change, and the force for maintenance of the status quo?

Parenting Ourselves

In facing our development head-on, we encounter challenge. One response is to plunge ahead, overriding any feelings of inadequacy, fear, or weakness. Another response is to decline the challenge: collapse, avoid, become ill. Between these two extremes, we are back on the developmental edge and reengaged in an internal dialogue. Negotiating this edge and dialoguing within ourselves can be seen as parenting ourselves. The development of an internal parent is a primary developmental task of adulthood.

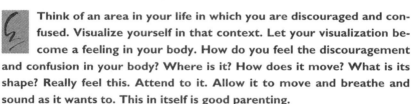

Think of an area in your life in which you are discouraged and confused. Visualize yourself in that context. Let your visualization become a feeling in your body. How do you feel the discouragement and confusion in your body? Where is it? How does it move? What is its shape? Really feel this. Attend to it. Allow it to move and breathe and sound as it wants to. This in itself is good parenting.

After you have established good contact with the feeling, notice how old this feeling seems to be. What is its age? Is the feeling infantile, childlike, or adolescent? Whatever the age, as the parent of this child, how would you care for it? What kind of love, support, and guidance does it need? Let yourself feel and imagine this love and support. Now ask yourself: "Am I willing to manifest this in my life?"

Often people misinterpret maturity to mean that one should be entirely self-sufficient. Parenting ourselves does not preclude receiving from others. In fact, one sign that we are successfully parenting ourselves is that we are able to accept love, guidance, and support from those outside us.

When we do not parent ourselves, we are struggling between the hope that someone else will take care of us and the fear that no one ever will. At the root of many adult life issues, I often find a little child waiting for his parents to grow up and parent him. More often than we care to admit, we allow our lives to manifest problems as a call for help: "Perfect mother, please come and fix this." On the one hand, it may be a hard reality to accept that it is up to us to live our lives. On the other hand, responsibility is wonderfully empowering. Utilizing the body can make parenting ourselves very concrete and graphic.

Parenting ourselves is an ongoing process that empowers us to guide and support ourselves without the illusion that we are in control. In the process of parenting ourselves, we are not following a predictable map; rather, we encounter lots of surprises along the way. Do we view these as obstacles or as opportunities?

WORKING WITH NEGATIVITY AND GENERATING BODILY WELL-BEING

When we view our lives as problematic and the events that arise as obstacles, we are creating negativity within ourselves. On an energetic level we are broadcasting a big "no." Biologically, that message means "Give up." Our cells hear this as a movement toward death. This is related to the freezing response of the lower brain which is also a biological aspect of the preparation for death. Whatever tissues and fluids are primarily involved with this response, they are immobilized into a very slow metabolic state. Occasionally this can be part of a healthy cycle of disorganization which is preparing for a new stage of evolution. However, habitually this becomes debilitating to one's physical and emotional health.

On a cognitive level, negativity arises when we are focused on what we don't have. This is very different from going toward what we want. In going toward what we want, we do not know if we are going to get there and we do not know what it is going to be like when we arrive. We do know what we want and that we are pursuing it. On a biological level, this is akin to aligning ourselves with life.

Negativity literally leaks physical energy. On a physical level, it renders satisfaction unlikely. On the other hand, the crudeness of "thinking positively" is simplistically offensive to some and can be seen as manipulative. Approaching well-being on a physical level, however, can ground positivity in reality. Consciously feel the parts of yourself that are saying "yes" to life. Allow them to move and breathe in their own way. When we restore a sense of well-being in our bodies and focus on a desirable direction in our cognition, productive and satisfying change can occur. The practice of generating well-being in the body involves breathing, moving, and listening to the messages of the body. Next time you are stuck in negativity, offer yourself this exercise.

Notice the repetitive thoughts you are using to maintain your negativity. You might be thinking, "This is horrible. I hate this. I can't. . . I won't . . ." There is almost always some mantra-like phrase we use to fixate in our negative state. Recognize this as the brain-washing it is. Breathe into your head with a sense of the insubstantiality of this thought. Be kind enough to yourself to feel the sensations in your body.

Give them permission to move and breathe in any way that is satisfying for them in that moment. Spend five or ten minutes with yourself in this way. Notice if there is a shift afterwards.

Generating well-being in the body cultivates fertile ground for creative experience. Well-being does not require that we be free of disease or physical disability, rather it requires circulation, breath, and a metabolism directed toward life and health.

Often, repetitive, subliminal negative messages block a sense of well-being. Despite breathing and moving, if messages like "I hate my life," "I'm not OK," or "This is horrible," are being broadcast, our basic metabolic direction is pointed toward death. Sometimes we cannot stop these negative movements toward death in our bodies. In this case, well-being might be a process of being kind to the negativity, washing it with fluids, supporting it with whatever developmental action might feel helpful, and reminding ourselves that it will pass.

Working with Our Cognitive Selves

Working with our cognition requires slowing down and becoming mindful. In this way we can hear our subliminal thoughts. We can take the time to test each thought for truthfulness and for helpfulness. If a thought is not true or not helpful, why think it? Thoughts powerfully affect our bodies right down to a cellular level. Thoughts that are affecting us negatively need to be worked through, debated, challenged, restated, or just plain discarded. Generally people try to discard them before actually hearing them out. This is usually ineffective. Often we may need to thoroughly debate them, extracting the truth or at least the essential intention. For example, a subliminal message of "You're lazy" could be dissected further. "Well, you're not lazy in these areas, but you're ignoring such and such." "Well, I'm ignoring that because I'm terrified of it, not because I'm lazy." At this point a helpful cognitive message might be something like "You're getting paralyzed by the terror again. Are you ready to touch this terror now. . . even just a little bit? . . . Breathe into it, let it move." The destructive thoughts need to be addressed and reworked.

Sometimes we know something in our brains but not in our bodies. Someone might say, "I know you care about me, but I feel like you hate me." Often when we "know" something or "believe" something, it has not been fully communicated to the rest of our body. It has not landed in the body systems or in the cells. This is often true with people suffering from post-traumatic stress disorder—though externally the war is over, no one has told the people living out in the hills. The message must be carried to each part of our physical being.

Pick a belief out of your own life, a belief that you "know" but you don't feel. Slow down; breathe. Let your brain rest downward. Often we subtly roll the front of our brains up and back in an effortful thinking pattern. Place the heels of your hands on your eyeballs. Imagine your brain rolling forward and feel its weight resting down, connecting into the rest of your body rather than pulling apart. Let your throat soften. In this way your brain's weight can yield down through your head and throat and rest into your trunk.

Think the thought you want to feel. Think it clearly and simply; use the first-person point of view. Rephrase any negative sentence constructions. For example, if the thought is "I don't want to fight anymore," rephrase it to say, "I want our relationship to be easy" or "I want to appreciate our differences." Find the way to say what is true without negative sentence construction. Also, simplify the sentence so that there are no clauses. We can only feel one thought at a time. Find the simplest version of the truth. Think it and breathe. Feel your bodily response. Where in your body is that thought free to travel? Where is it rebuffed? Keep breathing it where you want to send it. Feel the response as it arrives somewhere and then feel the response shift as it is absorbed on a cellular level.

A couple I worked with illustrates the need for communicating thoughts into specific parts of the body. Sue and Grant shared a great deal of love but very little sexual intimacy. They both felt a strong sexual drive, but did not share this with each other. In a session together, Sue, who had a history of sexual abuse, said that she wanted to be sexual with Grant. As she explored this statement she found that she felt that desire in her chest and throat and face, but it did not sequence below her diaphragm. It was as if her pelvis had not been informed of her desire. It had shut down with her abuse and had not received news of any other developments. Sue spent months consciously thinking about her husband, her sexuality, their love for each other, and intentionally breathing these thoughts down into her pelvis. As her pelvis began receiving this information, Sue was able to be sexual with Grant. As she continued breathing her news of her current life into her pelvis, the information began to be absorbed by the cells; she experienced mild cramping during her breathing sessions and some benign tissue discharge during her menstrual cycles. While these sensations were mildly uncomfortable, she was excited to be feeling more in her pelvis.

Our new experiences must be received by particular parts of the body to have particular effects. This directed communication is an important part of any kind of development, but it is of particular importance in a healing process.

The Healing Edge

Often the primary obstacles that we encounter in our development are attitudes and emotional responses that we have learned. Again, it is too easy to take a black-and-white view of these. Either we are stuck with these responses or they are so shrouded that we think they don't exist. Feeling our bodies brings reality to either of those two extremes. When we feel an emotion in our bodies, we can feel that it definitely exists—we cannot ignore it. However, we can also feel that it is moving. Even if that movement is only a tight throb, there is always movement in any sensation. By breathing and allowing the sensation to move as it wants to, it eventually sequences out, bringing us into a new position in the world. This may occur in a flash or over a long period of time.

Genuine healing occurs when we are feeling old pain and aware of a new possibility at the same time. I call this a healing edge. If we are just identified with the old pain, then we are just being retraumatized by it. But if there is some flickering awareness of our desire to heal and go beyond the limitations this old pain has engendered, then we are on a healing edge. We are bringing the past and the future together in the present moment. Dwelling solely on the past or solely on the future does not constitute healing. Bringing the past and future together in the present moment and feeling both pain and possibility in our bodies is a genuinely healing experience.

The Biological Basis of Emotions

When studying the behavior of animals, we do not speak of emotions. Instead, we see the functional aspect of their behavior. We see them asserting their territoriality, submitting to more powerful animals, avoiding danger, seeking food and water, nurturing their young, and bonding with their mates. These are the biological aspects of human emotion as well. It can be very helpful to remember these functional qualities when trying to understand a particular emotional response.

While there is always a limitation in formulas, particular emotions may have common patterns based on their function. Anger, for example, is based on defending one's territory. Thus, within the body, the energy of anger almost always needs to sequence out. Anger that does not sequence out is like an ingrown nail; it is only hurtful to the self. This does not mean that the anger must be pointed at someone else. By letting anger sequence out into space, we can discover the continuum between power and anger.

Barbara had learned early in life to turn her anger inward. Everything was all her fault. Her outlook was black and she was depressed in a furious way, not in a sad way but with great wrath. Often I would have to get her up off my office floor and have her mechanically begin the motions of angry gestures. Within minutes she was in touch with the fact that she was full of fury. Over time, Barbara, came to understand that there was tremendous energy underneath her depression, this state in which she felt that she could barely move. She also came to understand that berating her parents was never going to produce the love she wanted. Learning to reverse the habit of turning her anger inward developed slowly over a period of time. She choreographed an "angry" dance for herself, one that she danced frequently. This helped her learn about sequencing anger out. Slowly she began to learn to assert herself more.

In contrast to anger, sadness often requires a tender holding. Biologically, sadness is related to adjusting to loss, allowing our nervous systems to change familiar habits. Just as one holds a hurt bird, sadness must be held in a way that does not squash it but also does not abandon it. Often the root of sadness is pain that was left alone. In order to not perpetuate this pattern, take your sadness by the hand. Don't leave it at home alone. Bring it along, introduce it to your friends and love it until it runs out to play on its own. Often we check in on our sadness without the patience to really stay with it until it sequences through. If you must leave it, make a date with it to check back in. It is only a concept that we will cry forever or fall into an endless black hole. So many of us believe this and I have never found it to be true.

Biologically, our fear system is a very strong and powerful system designed to protect us from danger. Fear entails strong physiological responses that are often irrational. The primitive aspect of our brain recognizes the possibility of danger before we are able to accurately assess a situation. For example, when we see an object shaped like a snake, we may jump away quickly before we realized that it is a rope. That is our nervous system's way of saying, "Protect yourself first. Ask questions later." The physiological reactions to fear involve freezing, fighting, and fleeing. Therefore, once we recognize that the object is really a rope, there is already a strong physiological process in motion. To complete that cycle, animals let themselves shake, violently if need be. They embody the process of the fear and allow that cycle to complete itself.

As adult humans we often cut off that cycle without recognizing it. But pay attention next time you are afraid. Give your body permission to take care of itself. You might notice that fear often has a quivery quality. I recall reading a novel from the 1920s in which the character shook with fear. I was struck by the fact that people do not allow themselves to shake much these days. We hide our fear, masking our shakiness by freezing. Physically, fear needs to be acted on if there is real danger, or shaken off if it is an old fear or a false alarm. Rather than running from fear, breathe into it and let it shake and quiver until you realize either that you can act on the fear or that you are no longer afraid but excited by the new possibilities. Animals become alert at the possibility of danger, and when that is over, they shake the arousal off. When trauma has occurred in the life of a human being, a deep neurological arousal lingers in the more primitive parts of the brain. In releasing this from the body, often a very deep shudder begins at the base of the brain when the trauma response is integrated.

Moving Beyond the Boundaries of Our Familiar Selves

Whenever we grow beyond our habitual range, there is always some sort of sensory barrier acting as a fence to keep us from leaving our familiar pasture. Stan Grof (1988) coined the term *sensory barrier* from his encounters with transformation through breathwork. A sensory barrier might be dizziness, nausea, obsessive thinking, sleepiness, distractedness, or any sort of intense bodily sensation. This intensity is part of being alive in our bodies. Accepting intensity allows us to move through the sensory barrier, climb the fence, and explore new territory.

In order to become comfortable with our bodily sensations, we must learn to tolerate all sorts of energy, at many different levels of intensity. Energy is not good or bad—it is life force that can go in any direction. And it is always a package deal; good and bad unfold together. Many people who seek psychotherapy want lots of good things like love and joy, but they do not want to relate to challenging issues. All we can do is open up to aliveness and take what comes—healing and developing and transforming along the way.

Challenging Limiting Beliefs

Beyond emotional patterns, another aspect of life that can limit our growth are our beliefs. Both philosophy and science have taught us that beliefs are both relative and transient. But too often in our everyday life, we accept our beliefs, blindly, not pausing to consider whether or not they are true. Most of our beliefs are premature assumptions, generalizations, transient realities, or blatant falsehoods. Only the most basic and simplest experiences can be said to be experientially true: It is raining. I am typing.

Ferreting out, questioning, and disbanding beliefs can further one's pursuit of a developmental goal. Ask yourself frequently: "Is this thought or belief helpful to me in my development?" If it is not, can you let go of it or try a more productive approach?

Often our limiting beliefs take the form of the repetitive, negative thoughts that were discussed above. Other times, they are deeply hidden in our unconscious, exerting a powerful influence without ever being exposed. Going deeply into embodying our process through movement can unearth some of these thoughts. When you encounter pain or confusion in your body, ask yourself, "What is this part saying? Is there a message or a belief here?"

Limiting beliefs can also emerge as we move past the previous limits of our self. As we grow into a new aspect of our selves, limiting beliefs can arise to scare us back into the former confines of our old way of being. Messages may emerge such as "You'll get in trouble if you do that," or "You can't trust this," or "You're not really this way. You're just faking it." Limiting beliefs are one way in which our history solidifies itself into our future.

Choosing Our Histories

Our bodies are the most tangible record of ways in which our history has shaped us, and our bodies show us the ways in which we can move out of this shape into new possibilities. Engaging with ourselves at the cellular level of reality most clearly illustrates that we are not our histories. Engaging on a systemic and organismic level can reveal our old pattern or a new desire. Understanding our history and the emotional patterns and beliefs that it engendered can allow us to move beyond it. Tapping into the transformational quality inherent in cellular activity, we find that our bodies are fluid at the most fundamental level.

Expanding our repertoire always opens us to greater aliveness. Working with one's history requires a delicate touch, discriminating between what needs to be heard and felt from the past and what needs to be discarded. This is a process of human choice with no right and wrong. It can be guided by our intentions, but not controlled and predicted.

Working gently with ourselves to open to our own potential is a challenging path fraught with confusion, fear, and aggression. Our bodies can be the barometer for when to lean in and when to ease up. Bodies hold the paradoxical nature of being both extraordinarily real and earthy and grounded on the one hand, and holding tremendous potential to radically transform. May we tap into the deep spring of their natural intelligence.

Personal Inquiry and Exploration

The following exercise draws from the sections of this chapter involving desire, dialogue, and the developmental edge. Experiment with the whole thing or just focus on a part of it at a time.

- Take a moment to breathe and settle into your body.

- Contemplate how you have been struggling with reality lately in your life.

- Keep breathing and let that acknowledgment settle into a physical feeling of acceptance.

- From there, let yourself really contemplate what you are wanting in your life right now.

- As you think about this desire, really feel the parts of your body that open to the desire. Relax right into the idea. These are the parts of your body that are saying "yes" to that desire.

- Again feeling this desire, notice the parts of your body that are holding back from this, tensing up, shutting down. These are the parts of your body that are saying "no" to that desire.

- If there are particular locations in your body connecting the parts that are saying "yes" and the parts that are saying "no," you could shift your attention back and forth between the two. Breathe into each of them and the space in between them.

You might want to explore the following questions through writing.

- What kind of parent are you to yourself? How do you parent yourself in positive ways? If you could dream up the perfect parent for yourself right now, what kind of parent would that be? How can you embody this for yourself?

- Write about a recent time when you were stuck in negativity. Feel it in your body and imagine working with that feeling and generating well-being in your body. Write about how you would do that. This can become a model for the next time.

- What are limiting beliefs that you maintain about yourself?

- What are aspects of your history that you regret? Are you willing to begin to add to your history to go beyond these?

Awakening Natural Intelligence

There is a natural order and harmony to this world, which we can discover. But we cannot just study that order scientifically or measure it mathematically. We have to feel it—in our bones, in our hearts, in our minds.

—Chögyam Trungpa, Rinpoche

HAVING READ THE PRECEDING CHAPTERS AND EXPERIENCED THE EXERCISES, YOU MAY WANT TO GO FURTHER IN AWAKENING YOUR BODY'S INTELLIGENCE—ITS PERCEPTIVENESS, COMMUNICATIVENESS, AND RESPONSIVENESS. AS YOU AWAKEN THE SENSATIONS IN YOUR BODY, TWO BASIC ATTITUDES CAN HELP ENORMOUSLY—PERMISSION AND CURIOSITY. GIVING YOUR BODY PERMISSION TO DO WHAT IT WANTS TO DO, ALLOWING EACH SENSATION TO COMPLETE ITS PHYSIOLOGICAL TASK UNENCUMBERED, IS BOTH EMPOWERING AND ENERGIZING. HAVING CURIOSITY ABOUT THE INTELLIGENCE, THE MESSAGES, AND THE ONGOING DEVELOPMENTAL PROCESS IN WHICH YOUR BODYMIND IS ENGAGED, ALLOWS A HEALTHY INTERACTION BETWEEN THE COGNITIVE BRAIN AND THE REST OF YOU. USE THESE ATTITUDES—PERMISSION AND CURIOSITY—WHEN YOU FEEL STUCK OR IMPATIENT. IN THIS WAY, YOUR NATURAL INTELLIGENCE CAN UNFOLD IN ITS OWN UNIQUE MANNER.

✻   ✻   ✻

Modes of Inquiry

There are four primary modes of inquiry that you can use to continue your exploration into the body. These are moving, writing, contemplating, feeling, and sensing.

MOVE

The first step in deepening your relationship with your body is to spend more time with it—quality time in which there is no other agenda. I call this *moving* because that is what life does, it moves. On both a macroscopic and a microscopic level, there is constant movement in life. By calling this activity *moving*, I don't mean that you should be jumping around the whole time. Micromovements and internal physiological movements may be imperceptible to the outside eye.

Imagine the constant flow of activity through your body. Release yourself into that. Sometimes this might be large or loud. At other times it might be subtle and quiet. Review the suggestions in Chapter 2, "Natural Movement." Reread it again for inspiration. Set a specific amount of time for a period of moving, and then begin. Ask your whole bodymind, "Do you want to begin standing, sitting, or lying down?" and then check in with your sensations. Use a little bit of breath and a little bit of movement to help you scan through your body for sensations. Get a sense of an overall energy flow or map, and then let your attention shift as it naturally does. Wherever your attention goes, allow that sensation to move, breathe, and sound in its own way. If you find yourself thinking, observe how this thought feels in your body, and let yourself acknowledge those sensations.

Spending time like this every day can be one of the simplest ways to support overall health, get to know yourself better, and make basic changes in your life. Discover a rhythm that's right for you, whether it's once a day for fifteen minutes, three times a week for five minutes, whatever. Allow your attention span for your sensations to grow organically and your appetite for bodymind time will increase. Don't make this into a punitive activity in which you never reach your standards. Just observe your own interest and rhythm.

As you are curious, incorporate specific exercises into your natural movement time. This might include working with the endpoints, the basic actions or developmental movements from Chapter 4 , the body systems from Chapter 5, cellular explorations from Chapter 6, or more personal emotional experiments from Chapter 7. Reread these sections as you want to. My students are often amazed when they reread this material after working with it experientially. Their experience changes quite dramatically. Comments like "It's almost as if I've never read it before. I got so much out of it," are common.

You might have a friend who wants to practice some of the exercises from Chapter 3, "Embodied Relationship," with you. Spend time together practicing natural movement, and then explore one of the specific exercise, or see what happens if you both keep attending to your own bodies, as you move toward and away from each other.

Making noise can sometimes be an inhibiting issue. If you are concerned about making noises, tell your family, friends, or neighbors that you are working with some exercises from a book that involve making weird noises or animal sounds. Tell them whatever is needed so that you can both relax about it. Sometimes making noise is intimidating even if there's no one around to hear you. Start with listening to the sound of your exhalation. Make breathy noises that go out with your breath. Let those get louder and louder, just to experiment.

Be kind to any emotions that arise as you do this. Feel the specific sensations that carry them, and continue to allow those sensations permission to move, breathe, and sound however they like. Reread Chapter 7 if you need support with this.

And most importantly, enjoy! Notice how you feel after a session of natural movement. And if you are able to practice over a period of time, notice the changes in your body, your posture, your health, and your energy level.

WRITE

You may want to write after you move. You can write about what came up in your moving, specific sensations, images, memories, ideas, shifts in mood. You can write about your history with your body, your attitudes, what you learned from your family, your schooling, your culture. Write about the relationship you want with your body. Write about important dreams or events and notice how you feel and felt in your body in relationship to them. Write about how all this is integrating in your life.

CONTEMPLATE

At first, you might have the thought that you will never be able to integrate natural movement into your life. It might seem too socially unacceptable. This is true at first glance As you spend time moving, you often find yourself in strange positions, or making weird noises, or animal-like movements. Routinely, in working with this material in groups or classes, people laugh about this being an "insane asylum." Perhaps if we made more room for this sort of activity, we'd be less likely to lose our sanity.

However, after a while you might notice that you are feeling more sensations in a greater variety of situations. You might notice an interesting mutation. A sensation that might have led to some extreme movement during your movement practice becomes a slightly deeper breath in a formal social context. A slight push of your feet, a small shift in your spine, or a change in your breathing might be sufficient sequencing. You might find that you are able to allow your energy to continue to circulate freely even in extremely tense situations. You have become a master sequencer. Congratulations!

Contemplate any of the six principles of body-mind integration that seem challenging to you. Contemplation allows us to mix a simple thought with our moment-to-moment experience. For example, I have the word *breathe* on my computer screen saver. This reminds me at all sorts of interesting moments.

Set intentions for yourself and contemplate them throughout your day. Examples of this might be, "I want to feel my pelvis more," or "I want to push more through my hands to set boundaries." Contemplate them by repeating a simple reminder to yourself, "Pelvis," or "Push," and feel what happens in your body and in the situation.

FEEL AND SENSE

Notice your body in lots of different situations. Standing in line is a good time to practice noticing sensations and allowing them to sequence. Driving is a good time to feel your endpoints pushing and reaching. Check in with your body during emotionally charged moments—conflicts, ecstasy, boredom. If there are situations which chronically fatigue or overwhelm you, resolve to attend to your body a bit more next time.

Overall, enjoy the process, trust your pace, and notice the results.

My wish is that the ideas, stories, and tools in this book support you in your path toward body-mind integration and allow you to move toward greater aliveness. May we all stop underestimating the vast potential of the human body-mind. May we follow our bodies, as well as our minds, further and deeper into the emergence of our brilliant human animal. May we vibrate with life and overflow with our natural intelligence and compassion. May our culture integrate the natural intelligence of the human organism into a creative and sustainable lifestyle on this planet.

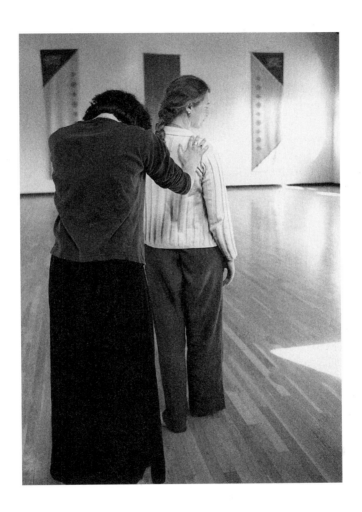

Glossary

body-mind dualism   ability to repress and ignore parts of ourselves which often results in opposing factions within our beings.

body-mind psychotherapy   approach to somatic psychotherapy developed by the author which integrates a deep experience of emotional and physical process down to a physiological level.

development   responsive, adaptive, and learning approach to living. One of the principles of body-mind integration.

dialogue   cooperative communication between parts and aspects of the bodymind. One of the principles of body-mind integration.

dissociation   term used in psychology to describe a lack of connection to one's body, one's feelings, and the present reality.

complete expressions   term coined by the British naturalist Charles Darwin (1809–1882) to contrast the responses of animals with the smaller, truncated gestures of humans. For example, the complete expression of a person's sneer might appear as snarling and baring of the incisors. Darwin believed that the full repertoire of animal movement that preceded us in evolution remains with us.

endpoints   major ports of the body through which information comes and goes, including the face, hands, pelvic floor, and feet, unique in several ways: skeletally, the endpoints are composed of many small bones with multiple joints; they are the free ends of the skeleton; muscularly, small muscles capable of precisely initiating and guiding movement compose the tissue of the endpoints; neurologically, they contain the highest concentration of sensory neurons in the body.

energetic development   process that correlates our emotional development with the actual movements we use to support ourselves and move toward and away from the external world.

experiential anatomy   approach to the study of anatomy in which one seeks to experience personally in one's own body the aspects of anatomy which are being explored.

full participation   empowerment of each aspect of the bodymind to shift in and out of initiatory and supportive roles as appropriate. One of the principles of body-mind integration.

inclusivity   cultivating participation by all parts and aspects of the bodymind. One of the principles of body-mind integration.

natural intelligence   synergistic intelligence that arises out of including all the resources of every tissue and fluid in the body down to the cellular level. Every system of the body has its own unique abilities to perceive and respond. For both cultural and evolutionary reasons, we ignore and override both sensory input and behavioral responses which arise outside the nervous system. Including and integrating the intelligence and creativity of the entire body is natural intelligence.

natural movement   1. phenomenon of spontaneously occurring movement characterized by a natural continuity between perception and sensation and movement whether this movement is large and visible, or the micromovement of minute shifting in the joints, or internal physiological movement; 2. practice of attending to sensations and allowing those sensations to move, breathe and sound in their own way.

neotony   term borrowed by biology from evolutionary theory to describe the quality of particular species in which certain qualities of infancy persist into adulthood

presence   degree to which every aspect of the bodymind is engaged in the present moment, including sensations, thoughts, and feelings.

respect   appreciation for the intelligence of the bodymind, its motivations, emotional tone, and responses. One of the principles of body-mind integration.

sequencing   uninhibited flow of energy within all parts and aspects of the bodymind and between ourselves and the environment. One of the principles of body-mind integration.

somatic psychology   field of psychological exploration which centers in the body. This field originated in the 1930 in the work of Wilhelm Reich.

Bibliography

Becker RO, Selden G. *The Body Electric*. New York: William Morrow, 1985.

Bohm D. *Quantum Theory*. New York: Prentice-Hall, 1951.

Cairns J, Overbaugh J, Miller S. Nature 1988;335:8,142–45.

Clark W. *Sex and the Origins of Death*. New York: Oxford University, 1996.

Campbell J. *The Power of Myth*. New York: Doubleday, 1988.

Cohen BB. *Sensing, Feeling and Action*. Northampton, Massachusetts: Contact Editions, 1993.

Eisler R. *The Chalice and the Blade*. San Francisco: Harper Collins, 1987.

Goldberg N. *Writing Down the Bones*. Boston: Shambhala Press, 1986.

Goodwin B. *How the Leopard Changed Its Spots*. New York: Charles Scribner's Sons, 1994.

Grof S. *Human Survival and Consciousness Evolution*. Albany, NY: State University of New York Press, 1988.

Hall SS. A molecular code links emotions, mind and health. Smithsonian Magazine 1989:62–71.

Harris RS, Longerich S, Roseberg SM. Science 1994;264:258–60.

Harlow H. Scientific American 1959;June.

Hendricks GK. *Conscious Breathing: Breathwork for Health, Stress, Release, and Personal Mastery*. New York: Bantam Books, 1995.

Iseman M. The Emotional/Psychological Aspects of the Basic Neurological Patterns,

Unpublished paper written in partial fulfillment of the certification program in Body-Mind Centering, 1989.

Jaynes J. *The Origin of Consciousness in the Breakdown of the Bicameral Mind*. Boston: Houghton Mifflin Company, 1976.

Kauffman S. *At Home in the Universe: The Search for the Laws of Self-Organization and Complexity*. New York: Oxford University Press, 1995.

Keleman S. *Emotional Anatomy*. Berkeley: Center Press, 1985.

Keleman S. *Your Body Speaks Its Mind*. Berkeley: Center Press, 1981.

Kordon C. *The Language of the Cell*. New York: McGraw-Hill, Inc, 1993.

Kurtz R. *Body-Centered Psychotherapy: The Hakomi Method*. Mendocino, California: LifeRhythm, 1990.

Levine P. *Waking the Tiger: Healing Trauma*. Berkeley: North Atlantic Books, 1997.

Lipton B. The Biology of Consciousness. Paper presented at the International Association for New Sciences, Fort Collins, Colorado, 1993.

MacLean P. *The Triune Brain in Evolution: Role in Paleocerebral Functions*. New York: Plenum Publishing Corporation, 1990.

McMenamin D, McMenamin M. *Hypersea*. New York: Columbia University Press, 1994.

McIntyre J. *Mind in the Waters*. New York: Charles Scribner's Sons, 1974.

Mead M. *Coming of Age in Samoa*. New York: Morrow Quill, 1961.

Mindell A, Mindell A. *Riding the Horse Backwards*. London: Arkana, 1992.

Montagu A. *Growing Young*. Westport, CT: Greenwood Publishing, 1989.

Moyers B. *Healing and the Mind*. New York: Doubleday, 1993.

Pert C. *Molecules of Emotion*. New York: Scribner, 1997.

Reich W. *Character Analysis*. New York: Touchstone, 1972;xi–481.

Satprem. *The Mind of the Cells*. New York: The Institute for Evolutionary Research, 1981.

Suzuki S. *Zen Mind, Beginner's Mind*. New York: Weatherhill, 1970.

Index

Page numbers in *italics* denote figures.